The Country Practitioner

The Country Practitioner

Ellis P. Townsend's Brave Little Medical Journal

Sandra W. Moss

Front cover: First issue of the *Country Practitioner* (courtesy University of Medicine and Dentistry of New Jersey, Special Collections)

To order additional copies of this book, contact:
Xlibris Corporation
1-888-795-4274
www.Xlibris.com
Orders@Xlibris.com
83155

CONTENTS

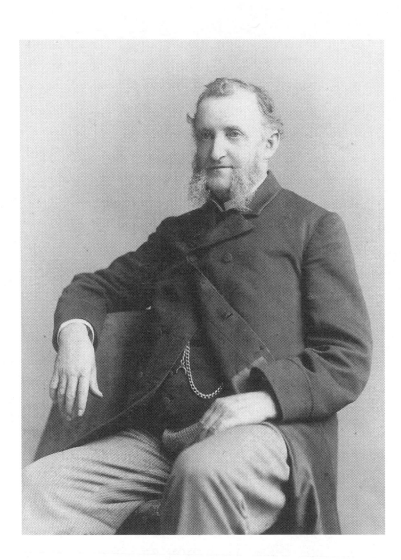

Ellis P. Townsend, M.D. (1835-1907). Photograph taken 1887 in Philadelphia. Property of Carol Townsend Oberweiser, granddaugher of Dr. Townsend, and published with her kind permission. Photograph made available by great-granddaughter Mary Oberweiser Andreoli and brought to the author's attention by great-grandniece René Delaney.

INTRODUCTION

When Dr. Ellis P. Townsend died in Montana in 1907, the *Journal of the American Medical Association* noted in his short obituary that he had been "at one time editor of a medical journal."[1] Between 1879 and 1881, while practicing as a physician in rural Burlington County, New Jersey, Townsend edited and published a unique and long-forgotten monthly journal called *The Country Practitioner; Or New Jersey Journal of Medical & Surgical Practice.* The preeminent historian of New Jersey medicine, David L. Cowen, characterized Townsend's journal as "lively," and indeed it was.[2] Copies of the *Country Practitioner* are not easy to find today. The only complete run known to exist in New Jersey is a photocopy at Special Collections at the University of Medicine and Dentistry of New Jersey, which also owns an original first issue.

Before turning to the *Country Practitioner* and its editor, Ellis P. Townsend, I briefly examine New Jersey's somewhat provincial medical landscape, the nature of rural medical practice in America, and pertinent aspects of medical journalism in the late-nineteenth century. Throughout, I have sought to locate Townsend and his journal in the medical climate of post-Civil War America.

As urban America expanded rapidly in the nineteenth century, the country doctor became more clearly distinct from his urban counterparts. Increasingly, American medical progress was linked to a rising contingent of elite urban specialists, many

---

[1]   "Obituary: Ellis P. Townsend," *Journal of the American Medical Association* 49 (1907): 710.

[2]   David L. Cowen, *Medicine and Health in New Jersey: A History* (Princeton: D. Van Nostrand, 1964), 60.

of whom held prestigious posts in medical colleges, dispensaries, and medical academies. These men dominated the American medical literature and transmitted the latest in European medical knowledge to the general practitioners in small-town and rural America. At the same time, rural practitioners remained wary of knowledge generated in big city hospitals and European clinics. American country practice and country patients were believed to have unique constitutions that mandated specific therapies. Similarly, country physicians considered themselves uniquely qualified by their own experience and that of physicians in similar practices to select the correct course of treatment for the individual patient.

A doctor working in relative isolation faced a host of practical problems unfamiliar to his city colleagues. Nineteenth-century American medical journals, most of them short-lived, were overwhelmingly urban in origin. In general, editors and most contributors were drawn from the urban elite. When Townsend presumed to publish and edit a medical journal from a small town in rural New Jersey, he led off the first issue with editorials addressing not only his fellow country doctors, but also the editors of major American journals. Townsend did not see the *Country Practitioner* merely as a new publication in a state sadly lacking in medical journals. Rather, he saw his audience as underserved rural and small-town physicians across the nation. Equally important, the *Country Practitioner* would give motivated practitioners a forum to present their own experience in practice as contributors to the national medical literature. The *Country Practitioner* was more than a "niche publication." It was in fact a specialty journal, much as family practice journals address a distinct specialty in medicine today.

Despite his limited goals and targeted audience, Townsend suffered the travails of all editors, scrambling for contributors as well as subscribers. His journal lasted for just twenty-seven monthly issues, not unusual for medical journals of the period. Townsend brought to his writing and editing his own experience as a country practitioner, and did his best to keep his subscribers up-to-date with advances in medical science and practice that he considered relevant. The *Country Practitioner* addressed a surprisingly broad range of contemporary issues. In articles and editorials, Townsend championed his favorite medications, gave forthright opinions on issues related to managing a medical practice, and spoke out on perennial problems such as licensure and quackery. Throughout this history, Townsend and his contemporaries speak, whenever possible, in their own voices. Physicians of the period did not shy away from strong opinions and tart prose. In the words of one subscriber, the *Country Practitioner* had "snap."

Townsend's professional life was also marked by "snap." His years as a New Jersey country practitioner were bracketed by professional adventures in locales ranging from Gettysburg to the deep Amazon and finally to a Cheyenne reservation in rural Montana.

ACKNOWLEDGEMENTS

I am grateful to Vincent Cirillo, Lois Densky-Wolff, Gerald Grob, Alan Lippman, Karen Reeds, and Robert Vietrogoski for their comments on various drafts of this history. The expert assistance of archivists at the University of Medicine and Dentistry of New Jersey (Special Collections), Rutgers University Archives and Special Collections, the Montana State Historical Society, and the Burlington County (New Jersey) Historical Society is gratefully acknowledged. René Delaney, a great-grandniece of Ellis P. Townsend generously shared her painstaking genealogical research. Chris Becker provided expert assistance as copyreader. Portions of earlier drafts of this paper were presented at meetings of the American Osler Society, Cleveland, OH (2009), the University of Medicine and Dentistry of New Jersey—New Jersey Medical School, Newark, NJ (2010), and the Medical History Society of New Jersey (2010).

NOTE ON REFERENCES

Abbreviations are used as follows in footnotes: *CP* (*Country Practitioner*), EPT or [EPT] (signed or [assumed] authorship by Ellis P. Townsend), *TMSNJ* (*Transactions of the Medical Society of New Jersey*). Because of its central place in this history and the rarity of extant copies of the *County Practitioner*, the issue number and month of publication are given with each citation.

CHAPTER 1

AMERICAN MEDICAL JOURNALISM:
A PLACE FOR NEW JERSEY?

Medical articles and case reports by Americans in the mid-nineteenth century were, on the whole, written by physicians who made their living through private medical practice; of these, the vast majority were general practitioners. The journal editors themselves were also active practitioners. As the century progressed, specialists and the published transactions of their fledgling specialty societies were increasingly evident in the American medical landscape. Medical school professors, who were frequent contributors to medical journals, were first and foremost active practitioners, albeit with a predominately urban and often well-to-do clientele. In some cases, they used their part-time volunteer posts as consultants to infirmaries and charity hospitals as a means to enhance their medical knowledge, gain useful practical experience, and record interesting cases. Their medical school appointments, however prestigious, were part-time and often constituted a negligible portion of their income. There were no full-time researchers; research was undertaken as a private pursuit of motivated practitioners when time and the demands of practice permitted.[1] Research papers and monographs

---

[1]   W. Bruce Fye, "Medical Authorship: Traditions, Trends, and Tribulations," *Annals of Internal Medicine* 113 (1990): 317-19.

were published independently, outside the university or medical college framework.

Typically, nineteenth-century American medical journals featured case reports, state-of-the-art review articles, original articles, transcriptions of lectures from medical schools, summaries of the proceedings of professional organizations such as the New York Academy of Medicine, local and state medical society transactions, correspondence, book reviews, and editorials.[2] In addition many journal editors freely reprinted articles from other journals, both American and European; such articles were usually credited with the name of the journal from which they were taken, although volume and page were often omitted. In some journals, summaries of selected articles from American and European medical journals were included in a separate section. The average American general practitioner had relatively little interest in the scientific output of European laboratories and institutes, preferring the practical writings of his own countrymen.[3] At a time when there were few medical libraries or academies outside major cities and most practitioners subscribed to few, if any, journals, such reprinting or summarizing of articles from other journals was a legitimate way of disseminating information (or disinformation). Editors across the country exchanged complimentary copies of each issue; it was from such journal exchanges that many reprinted articles were taken.

The greatest challenge for medical editors was filling the pages of their monthly or quarterly publications. Editors routinely appealed (and in some cases, begged) for submissions. The need for publishable articles far exceeded the supply.[4] It is also important to recall that many American physicians lacked preparatory education beyond high school (or the much-abused "equivalent"), and some were marginally literate. Charles W. Eliot, the Harvard president who brought the medical school under the university's umbrella, remarked in 1869, that "hundreds of

---

[2] W. Bruce Fye, "The Literature of American Internal Medicine: A Historical View," *Annals of Internal Medicine* 106 (1987): 453-55.

[3] Ibid., 457.

[4] Fye, "Medical Authorship," 318.

young men joined the medical schools who could barely read and write . . . ."[5]

The foremost expert on American medical writing and publications was John Shaw Billings, a young and undistinguished surgeon with a genius for archival work. In 1865, he began assembling and organizing the medical literature, both American and international, for the Library of the Surgeon-General of the United States Army. By 1895, Billings had built the Surgeon-General's Library into the world's largest repository of medical literature. Over the course of three decades, from the 1860s to the 1890s, he undertook the monumental task of compiling and editing a comprehensive guide to the journal articles and other works included in the collection. The sixteen-volume first series of *The Index-Catalogue of the Library of the Surgeon General's Office, United States Army*, was published between 1880 and 1895. Billings' biographer called the *Index-Catalogue* "a bibliographic instrument of immense scope and unmatched usefulness to workers in the biosciences . . . ."[6]

In 1876 and again in 1879, Billings found time to review the history and current status of American medical journalism. His assembled data was precise and his comments were blunt; he did not consider America's late start an excuse for poor quality. The majority of nineteenth-century medical journals lasted just a few years, some just a few issues. Quality, wrote Billings, varied from excellent to terrible—"as bad as, but not worse than, the worst" of the foreign medical journals. Minor journals, in Billings' view, were prone to accepting articles by men with

> . . . defective mental training and an inability to comprehend the relations of the facts that are known, the result of which is a stringing out of a series of irrelevant and tedious details . . . .

5   Quoted in Florence Rena Sabin, *Franklin Paine Mall—The Story of a Mind* (Baltimore: Johns Hopkins University Press, 1934), 20; no primary source given.

6   Carleton B. Chapman, *Order Out of Chaos: John Shaw Billings and America's Coming of Age* (Boston: Boston Medical Library, 1994), 171. The collection of books and journals assembled by Billings was the nucleus of the present National Library of Medicine. *The Index-Catalogue* is fully searchable online through the National Library of Medicine's website. The fifth and last series of the *Index-Catalogue* was completed in 1961.

Many articles intended to be practical, are very far from being such, although the authors would probably be surprised and indignant to hear them termed otherwise.[7]

Billings did not hesitate to suggest that the editors of many minor journals had self-serving motives—although financial gain was rarely, if ever, expected or realized. In some cases, the editor/practitioner used his journal as a vehicle for self-promotion—a means of getting his name before the profession without violating the strict anti-advertising code of ethics of the American Medical Association.[8] More common, in Billings' somewhat cynical view, was the launching of a minor journal by an editor who sought a bully pulpit, "a place in which [he] can speak his mind and attack his enemies without restraint."[9]

The first American journal specifically aimed at physicians was the *Medical Repository*, published in New York from 1797 to 1824. According to Billings, as of the Centennial year of 1876, New York State had been, at one time or another, home to over fifty medical journals (most short-lived), as well as eleven current journals.[10] Billings identified thirty-one medical journals originating in New York City.[11] Pennsylvania had over twenty-five journals prior to 1879, many relatively short-lived, while others were renamed or merged.[12] Philadelphia was home to at least

---

[7] John Shaw Billings, "Literature and Institutions," in Edward H. Clarke, Henry J. Bigelow, Samuel D. Gross, T. Gaillard Thomas, J.S. Billings, *A Century of American Medicine 1776-1876* (Philadelphia: Henry C. Lea, 1876; repr. New York: Burt Franklin, 1971), 339, 341.

[8] American Medical Association, *Code of Medical Ethics of the American Medical Association*, (Chicago: American Medical Association Press, 1847), 98. Full text of the 1847 *Code of Medical Ethics of the American Medical Association* is reproduced online at http://www.ama-assn.org/ama1/pub/upload/mm/369/1847code.pdf (accessed July 2, 2010). The section on advertising appears in chapter 2, article 1, paragraph 3: "It is derogatory to the dignity of the profession, to resort to public advertisements or private cards or handbills, inviting the attention of individuals afflicted with particular diseases."

[9] J[ohn] S[haw] Billings, "The Medical Journals of the United States," *Boston Medical and Surgical Journal* 100 (1879): 2.

[10] Billings, "The Medical Journals of the United States," 7-9; Billings, "Literature and Institutions," 331-32.

[11] Billings, "Literature and Institutions," 331-32.

[12] Billings, "Medical Journals of the United States," 10.

seven journals, beginning with the *Philadelphia Medical Museum*, published from 1804 to 1811. The most important and prestigious of Philadelphia's extant journals was the *American Journal of the Medical Sciences*, founded in 1820. Billings considered this the premier American medical publication of his day, with its "original papers of the highest value; nearly all the real criticisms and reviews which we possess, and . . . carefully prepared summaries of the progress of medical science, and abstracts and notices of foreign works . . . ."[13]

Despite the absence of medical schools, teaching hospitals, medical libraries, and prestigious scientific academies, New Jersey physicians, both rural and urban, saw themselves as participants in, or at least beneficiaries of, a new scientific medicine. Insisted one leading New Jersey physician in 1888, "There is no medical wilderness between New York and Philadelphia."[14] Wilderness or not, New Jersey's contribution to the national medical literature was modest in the extreme and strictly provincial. With the founding of the Medical Society of New Jersey in 1766, the record of the society's transactions, including papers read at meetings and discussions of medical topics, were preserved but not published. In 1847, Joseph Parrish, a Philadelphian who practiced for some years in the city of Burlington, New Jersey, founded the *New Jersey Medical Reporter and Transactions of the New Jersey Medical Society* (from 1856, the *New Jersey Medical and Surgical Reporter*), publishing and editing it until 1856 from Burlington. From 1856 to 1858, the editor was S.W. Butler, who published from both Burlington and Philadelphia. In 1858, all operations were transferred to Philadelphia, where the journal continued as the more prestigious *Medical and Surgical Reporter* and lost all

---

13   Billings, "Literature and Institutions," 332-33.
14   Ezra Mundy Hunt, "Origin of Disease and Micro-Organisms as Related Thereto," *TMSNJ* (1888): 110. Hunt was New Jersey's leading public health advocate and reformer. Although left purposely vague by Hunt, the deprecating remarks were probably in response to comments made by Dowling Benjamin of Camden to the effect that there were only two physicians in New Jersey who accepted the germ theory in the mid 1860s, followed by comments about Hunt's tardiness in embracing the germ theory. Benjamin Dowling, "The Present Position of Antiseptic Practice," *TMSNJ* (1887): 253.

connections to New Jersey.[15] In 1859, the annual *Transactions of the Medical Society of New Jersey,* a collection of unedited essays and case reports, notes of county correspondents on prevailing diseases, and society business, began annual publication.[16]

Issues of quality and quantity aside, the contrast in intellectual ferment between New York and Pennsylvania on the one hand, and New Jersey on the other, was striking. The paucity of local medical publications could in no way be blamed on a widespread urge among New Jersey doctors to publish in more prestigious journals based in Philadelphia and New York. Contributions to publications such as the *Medical Record* (New York) or the *American Journal of the Medical Sciences* (Philadelphia), even at the rudimentary level of the case report, were confined to a mere handful of New Jersey physicians.

With the founding of the Country Practitioner in 1879, Ellis P. Townsend stepped into this rather turbulent world of American medical journalism. He imagined an audience of rural and small-town general practitioners across the nation—men who faced common problems that set them aside from their urban colleagues. He saw such general practitioners as underserved by the major publications and believed that they would be inspired to contribute articles to a journal aimed at men like themselves, free from real and perceived intimidation from the professional elite of the big American cities.

---

[15]   Billings, "Medical Journals of the United States," 7.

[16]   In 1875, at the behest of the Medical Society of New Jersey, Dr. Stephen Wickes of Essex County edited the collection of minute books and loose papers from 1766 to 1858 and assembled them into a single volume. Stephen Wickes, ed., *The Rise, Minutes, and Proceedings of the New Jersey Medical Society, Established July 23rd, 1766* (Newark: Jennings and Hardham, 1875). *The Transactions of the Medical Society of New Jersey* (1859-1904) was succeeded by the edited *Journal of the Medical Society of New Jersey*; the journal was renamed *New Jersey Medicine* in 1985. It ceased publication in 2005, leaving New Jersey with no state medical journal.

CHAPTER 2

WHAT DID COUNTRY DOCTORS WRITE AND WHAT DID THEY WANT TO READ?

In 1868, prominent New York medical editor George Shrady remarked upon the growing interest in country practice among medical graduates. Country doctors, insisted Shrady, deserved respect: The "metropolitan doctor" can no longer patronize his "rustic brother," and erstwhile "scoffers" are "prepared to study with profit the distinguishing traits of the country physician's character." Patients of the new country doctor, Shrady continued, were daily reaping the benefits: " . . . the veriest backwoodsman is being blessed with all the recent improvements that the advancement of science has beneficently showered upon the healing art."[1]

It was generally acknowledged that setting up in urban practice was a long and uncertain endeavor for those without professional or family connections. For example, John Sedgwick Billings, the son of John Shaw Billings, found that patronage and the best medical training the United States had to offer did not guarantee success among New York's fiercely competitive medical elite in the 1890s.[2] For many young and well-trained

---

[1] [George Shrady], "The Country Practitioner," *Medical Record* (New York) 3 (1868): 229-30. Shrady, as editor, is presumed to be the author of this unsigned editorial. Historian of medicine W. Bruce Fye drew my attention to Shrady's editorial.

[2] Charles E. Rosenberg, "Making It in Urban Medicine: A Career in the Age of Scientific Medicine," in *Explaining Epidemics and Other Studies in the History of*

medical graduates, country and small-town practice beckoned. The stereotypical "old fogy" and his outdated therapeutic regimens were fading away.[3] New technologies such as the ophthalmoscope and the laryngoscope were making their way out from the urban centers. Physicians everywhere were expected to be familiar with applied diagnostic technologies such as stethoscopic examination and urinalysis. For Shrady, the country doctor epitomized Yankee self reliance: "To be a reliable country practitioner, one equal to every ordinary emergency, calls for fully as much if not more preparation than is required of the mass of our physicians in the cities." The country doctor was, of necessity, required to be his own apothecary and very often his own consultant. He stayed longer at the bedside than the harried city doctor, observing the progress of his patient and the effects of his therapy. Overstating the case somewhat, Shrady added:

> . . . our periodicals teem with wise suggestions and original observations from their [i.e., country doctors'] pens, and many a physician who writes from the wilds of our territories, whose yearly income would hardly pay the driving expenses of some of our metropolitans, and whose patients are only backwoodsmen, is rapidly gaining an enviable and enduring reputation.[4]

Medical historian W. Bruce Fye, in a 1989 paper, asked, "Why do practitioners write?" Fye's answers apply equally well to nineteenth-century physicians, both urban and rural, as to the late-twentieth-century audience he was addressing. Of course, some practitioners, whether they read the medical journals or not, had no interest in, or aptitude for, preparing and submitting articles to medical journals. In nineteenth-century New Jersey, most physicians were content with the occasional paper read before their local or county medical societies. Motivating factors for the

---

Medicine (Cambridge: Cambridge University Press, 1992), 215-42.

[3]   [Shrady], "Country Practitioner," 229. The term "old fogy" was also used in a more light-hearted commentary by EPT on the subject of young men trying to set up practice; [EPT], "Practice Hunters," *CP* 2, no. 11 (April 1881): 366-67.

[4]   [Shrady], "Country Practitioner," 230.

physician who *did* want to write and publish articles included a desire to expand knowledge, a need to affirm the value of his professional work, and a calculated effort to boost his reputation among colleagues and elite patients.[5] No doubt many physicians were gratified, then as now, by seeing their names in print, an immodest but perfectly understandable and not unseemly sentiment. There is no reason to think that motivated country doctors, despite their paucity of glittering credentials, differed from upper echelon urban physicians in their reasons for writing and publishing, although the urban elite were probably under greater pressure to keep their names before the profession.

What did the country doctor need and want to read in a medical journal? Medical authority based on bedside experience, rather than laboratory science or clinical research, was still highly valued in post-Civil War America. The observations of elite European or American physicians with city practices and access to large urban hospitals were not necessarily considered superior to the observations of a seasoned general practitioner in rural or small-town practice. Nor were the therapies touted by urban physicians *a priori* applicable to country practice. It was an axiom of American medicine that country dwellers, blessed with fresh air and obliged to perform invigorating outdoor work, possessed constitutions distinctly different from those of the denizens of crowded cities, who breathed vitiated air in sunless factories and tenements. American practitioners clung to the concept that correct treatment required knowledge of the circumstances of the individual patient, including such factors as temperament, constitution, gender, race and ethnicity, region of habitation, climate, occupation, diet, habits, and family tendencies.[6] The country doctor, in short, sought practical guidelines, particularly those written by physicians from his own region, who dealt with similar kinds of patients living in similar climates and circumstances.

---

[5] Fye, "Medical Authorship," 317-18.
[6] John Harley Warner, "From Specificity to Universalism in Medical Therapeutics: Transformation in the 19th-Century United States," in *Sickness and Health in America*, 3rd ed., eds. Judith Walzer Leavitt and Ronald L. Numbers (Madison: University of Wisconsin Press, 1997), 88-91.

Ellis P. Townsend, the future editor of the *Country Practitioner*, practiced medicine in a small town in New Jersey's Burlington County for almost fifteen years before bringing out his new journal in 1879. His father, with whom he served an apprenticeship, had been a general practitioner in rural Pennsylvania for many years. In 1881, Townsend assured the readers of his journal that he understood how difficult country practice could be, noting that he himself had been "under fire for eighteen years," and was a practical rather than a theoretical man.[7] Townsend's experience in practice determined the unique direction his journal would take.

---

[7]   [EPT], "Editorial," *CP* 2, no. 2 (May 1881): 423. Townsend opened his practice in Beverly in 1864, accounting for fifteen years in country practice when he founded his journal in 1879. His figure of eighteen years, given in 1881, dated from his graduation from medical school in 1863 and included his year of military practice in the Civil War.

CHAPTER 3

EARLY YEARS IN BEVERLY: THE BURDENS AND REWARDS OF GENERAL PRACTICE

Southern New Jersey's sprawling Burlington County was sparsely settled and predominantly rural. The 1875 report from the Burlington County Medical Society to the Medical Society of New Jersey noted that Burlington County was the largest in the state (six hundred square miles) and was third in population.[1] Members of the Burlington County Medical Society, scattered across the county, numbered twenty-three in that year. For comparison, populous Essex County, with its chief city of Newark, claimed fifty-three members.[2]

The town of Beverly, some fifteen miles up the Delaware River from Philadelphia, was known in Colonial days as Dunk's Ferry. Located a few miles south of the city of Burlington (county seat and former capital of West Jersey), Beverly covered less than a square mile. George Washington visited the town during

---

[1]   S.C. Thornton, "Reports of County Societies: Burlington County," *TMSNJ* (1875): 113.

[2]   "Members of District Societies," *TMSNJ* (1875): 6, 8. The population of Essex County in 1880 was approximately 190,000 and the population of Burlington County at that date was approximately 55,000, according to the New Jersey State Data Center, "New Jersey Resident Population by County: 1880-1920," in *New Jersey Population Trends: 1790-2000* (Trenton: New Jersey Department of Labor, 2001), 23, http://lwd.dol.state.nj.us/labor/lpa/census/2kpub/njsdcp3.pdf (accessed August 26, 2010).

the Revolutionary War, a fact considered worthy of note by local historians. Beverly was incorporated as a borough in 1850 and as a city in 1859. The population of Beverly and the surrounding villages (comprising Beverly Township) in 1880 was between seventeen and eighteen hundred. A regional history lists six physicians who served the town and undoubtedly the surrounding countryside prior to 1883. A man referred to only as Dr. Warren in one county history was the first resident physician and pharmacist. "Warren" was probably Justin Bliss Warriner, M.D., who died during a cholera epidemic in 1849 at the age of thirty-one, a mere two months after arriving in Beverly from Burlington City.[3] He was followed by Dr. William Bryan and later his son John W. Bryan, and a Dr. Trimble.[4] The tenure and years of overlap of these physicians are unknown.

Ellis P. Townsend, M.D., aged twenty-nine, arrived in Beverly in 1864. As of 1866, there were four physicians in Beverly, of whom Townsend alone was a member of the county society.[5] According to a local historian, he was descended from a long line of West Chester (Pennsylvania) Quakers. Townsend was born May 25th, 1835, in Kennett (Chester County), about twenty-five miles southwest of Philadelphia.[6] He served a medical apprenticeship with his father, William W. Townsend, M.D., and graduated from the two-year course at Jefferson Medical College in Philadelphia in 1863. His father had graduated from the same school in 1844.[7] Townsend's entry into medical school after the outbreak of the

---

[3]   Nancy M. Wade, "Historic Homes and Genealogy," in *Beverly: A Local History*, ed. Paragraph Club (Beverly: Paragraph Club and Beverly Bicentennial Committee, 1977), 121.

[4]   W.H. Shaw, "Beverly Township and City," in E.M. Woodward and John F. Hageman, *History of Burlington and Mercer Counties* (Philadelphia: Everts and Peck, 1883), 239.

[5]   "Regular Physicians in New Jersey: 1866," *TMSNJ* (1866): 313. The other three Beverly physicians were John W. Bryan, Wm. Bryan, and Wm. M. Woolsey.

[6]   Wade, "Historic Homes and Genealogy," 128.

[7]   John R. Stevenson, "A History of Medicine and Medical Men," in *A History of the Camden County Medical and Surgical Society*, ed. George R. Prowell (Philadelphia: L.J. Richards, 1886), 294; Frederick B. Wagner, Jr. and J. Woodrow Savacool, eds., *Thomas Jefferson University: A Chronological History and Alumni Directory, 1824-1990* (Philadelphia: Thomas Jefferson University, 1992), 773. http://jdc.jefferson.edu/cgi/viewcontent.cgi?article=1032&context=wagner1 (accessed July 2, 2010).

Civil War and his military service as a physician in 1863 suggests that his Quaker sensibilities may have prompted him to serve as a physician rather than as a combatant.

Some years later, Townsend reminisced about his first call as a young medical graduate in the Pennsylvania town in which his father was in practice. He was summoned in the middle of the night to the bedside of a "leading lady of the neighborhood." Since the patient herself was "apparently insensible," he took a detailed but utterly confusing history from family members. Unsure of what to do (and terrified of losing his very first patient), he "finally lit upon the happy idea of sending six miles through darkness, mud and mire, and dragging [his] invalid father from his midnight slumbers to aid [his] diagnosis." The senior Townsend quickly diagnosed "hysteroidal troubles" (a pattern of hysterical behavior) and administered a "stout" dose of valerian, a popular sedative, with excellent results.[8]

Shortly after earning his medical degree, Townsend served one year in the Union army as an assistant surgeon. He was posted to Camp Letterman General Hospital, a massive tent hospital set up under the direction of Dr. Jonathan Letterman, medical director of the Army of the Potomac, to care for thousands of Union and Confederate wounded. The hospital opened in mid-July, 1863, two weeks after the Battle of Gettysburg and was decommissioned and closed in November, 1863. By Civil War standards, it was a properly organized, if overtaxed, facility.[9] *The Medical and Surgical History of the War of the Rebellion*, an exhaustive multivolume review of army medical activities, indexes Dr. E.P. Townsend and locates him at the Letterman Hospital between July 3rd, 1863, and November 5th, 1863, where he participated in the care of the wounded men, both Union and Confederate. Listed under Townsend's name in the index of *The Medical and Surgical History*

---

[8]   EPT, "Medical Heroism" *TMSNJ* (1876): 97-98. This would have taken place either immediately following graduation and prior to his military service or, possibly, in a short interval between the end of military service and his arrival in Beverly. Valerian was a herbal preparation used to treat disorders of the nervous system including epilepsy, neuralgia, and hysteria. Henry Beasley, *The Book of Prescriptions* (Philadelphia: Lindsay & Blakiston, 1857), 357.

[9]   National Park Service, "Camp Letterman General Hospital," www.nps.gov/archive/gett/getttour/sidebar/letterman.htm; (accessed June 24, 2010).

were several pathological specimens sent to the Army Medical Museum in Washington. Townsend may have conducted the autopsies himself or, more likely, functioned as a junior assistant to more experienced men.[10] How much latitude he was given in attending to living patients is unknown, but many young medical graduates were plunged into Civil War work with little preparation. Since Camp Letterman Hospital was comparatively well-organized and staffed, it is likely that senior surgeons provided Townsend with some measure of supervision.

Details of the rest of Townsend's military service are lacking. He did not serve for the duration, but settled into civilian practice in Beverly in 1864. His reason for choosing Beverly is unknown, but several factors may have played a role in his choice of the small town on the Delaware. His father, William W. Townsend, had served in the Civil War military hospital at Beverly as an assistant surgeon in 1863. The makeshift hospital was housed in a converted building of the Baumgardner Cordage Works. Sick and wounded were transported by boat or train and some one hundred and forty military men were buried in the military cemetery in the course of the war. There is no evidence that Ellis P. Townsend served in the hospital.[11] A report of forty-five "capital" surgical operations performed at the hospital between August, 1864, and March, 1865, names several surgeons, but neither William W. nor Ellis P. Townsend was among them.[12] There is evidence, however, that the younger Townsend had some relationship to the hospital without an actual staff appointment; at an April, 1865, meeting of the Burlington County Medical Society, he "presented for the

[10]   Office of the Surgeon General, *Medical and Surgical History of the War of the Rebellion* (Washington: Government Printing Office, 1870-1888; repr. with editorial additions, Wilmington NC: Broadfoot Publishing Co., 1990); entries for Ellis P. Townsend: 9:372, 11:79, 11:186, 12:436, 12:530.

[11]   W.W. Townsend, EPT's father, graduated from Jefferson Medical College in 1844; *Medical Directory of Philadelphia, Pennsylvania, and Delaware and the Southern Half of New Jersey* (Philadelphia, P. Blakiston, Son & Co., 1885), 248. W.W. Townsend's service in Beverly during the Civil War is confirmed in Samuel W. Butler, ed., *The Medical Register and Directory of the United States* (Philadelphia: Office of the Medical and Surgical Reporter, 1878), 696.

[12]   C[linton] Wagner, *Report of Interesting Surgical Operations Performed at the U.S.A. General Hospital, Beverly, New Jersey* (1865). Photocopy courtesy American Philosophical Society, Philadelphia.

inspection of the members, a portion of the colon, taken from a post mortem made at the Beverly Hospital."[13]

It is also possible that the Townsends had relatives in Burlington County, as many Pennsylvania Quakers had family connections in southern New Jersey. However, an unconfirmed genealogical source claims that Townsend was disowned by the Quakers for serving in the military and for marrying "out of unity" (i.e. to a non-Quaker), suggesting that his marriage may have prompted him to move away from his birthplace.[14] He married Almira "Jennie" Johnston (b. 1839), formerly a schoolteacher in Lancaster, Pennsylvania, in 1861, the year he entered medical college.[15] The need to make a living was pressing. One, and possibly two, children were born during the Civil War, neither of whom survived infancy. The first surviving child, a son, was born in 1865.[16]

Beverly, ideally situated for a country retreat for well-to-do Philadelphians and Burlingtonians, was a town set to grow in the decade after the Civil War. By 1874, there were over one hundred and forty private homes in Beverly, some fronting on the river. The town also boasted five churches, one oilcloth factory, a

---

[13] *Secretary's Book: Burlington County Medical Society: 1829-1868* (entry April 1865); Burlington Country Medical Society Records, University Libraries Special Collections, University of Medicine and Dentistry of New Jersey, Newark, NJ.

[14] Richard Cramer, "Ellis P. Townsend: 1835-1907," Genealogy.com website, http://genforum.genealogy.com/townsend/messages/481.html (accessed June 20, 2010). The information about Townsend's expulsion from the Quaker meeting was posted by Richard Cramer in 1991 and could not be confirmed; the website is inactive.

[15] Delaney, René, "Genealogy: Ellis P. Townsend + Almira Jennie Johnston," PhpGedView website, http://renesfamily.com/family/family.php?famid=F00439&ged=Renes. GED (accessed July 2, 2010). Genealogical information on this webpage is well documented.

[16] Ibid., The site lists seven children, including the four surviving children named in the 1880 census. It is assumed that three children died at birth or in early childhood. Original worksheets used by census takers for 1880 and other census years are reproduced on Ancestry.com. A second (inactive) genealogy site, which lacks documentation, lists eight children, the first born in 1862 and dying in early childhood; Cramer, http://genforum.genealogy.com/townsend/messages/481.html (accessed September 9, 2010). Family records of René Delaney record an "unknown Townsend" as the first child born to the couple, although the date and place of birth is not recorded.

cordage factory, a cotton factory, and a steam sash and planing (lumber processing) mill.[17]

Townsend, who participated actively in community affairs, was characterized by a local historian as a "colorful figure in Beverly's history."[18] During his first few years in practice, he had time on his hands. By his own account, he was averaging fewer than one medical call daily during his third year in practice; the first two years were probably even leaner.[19] From 1866 to 1867, he served the Beverly municipal government as assessor; this post may have provided a modest salary. His civic duties extended into the 1870s; in 1872, for example, he was authorized by the district to purchase a large lot of land as a site for a future school.[20]

A decade after he arrived in Beverly, Townsend wrote a pamphlet entitled *Suburban Homes*. Apparently something of a booster and real-estate promoter, Townsend sought to attract wealthy citizens from Philadelphia to the bucolic town graced with elegant homes. In his text, generously embellished with the names of leading local citizens and seasonal visitors, he boasted that the "entire shore is now adorned with beautiful and costly cottages and mansions." He rhapsodized about the view from the river ("no more beautiful landscape can be seen in America" at sunset on a summer evening) and the "delightful homes, such as men dream of, and oft build in airy castles, but seldom realize."[21]

Physicians across New Jersey routinely praised the health of their localities, from the Atlantic shore through the Pine Barrens and into the hills of Essex County.[22] Townsend, citing his ten years

---

[17]   Wade, "Historic Homes and Genealogy," 131 *passim*.

[18]   Wade, "Historic Homes and Genealogy," 128.

[19]   EPT, "Tabular Statement of Diseases Occurring in the Practice of Dr. E.P. Townsend, Beverly, N.J., January, 1868 to January, 1869," *TMSNJ* (1869): 126.

[20]   Shaw, "Beverly Township and City," 231, 245.

[21]   EPT, *Suburban Homes*, (ca. 1874), 1-3. No further details of publication are given in the pamphlet; photocopies courtesy Burlington County Historical Society. An outline of the contents of the pamphlet and a date of 1874 is in Wade, "Historic Homes and Genealogy," 128-31.

[22]   For a discussion of local meteorological boosterism in nineteenth-century New Jersey, see Sandra W. Moss, "The Doctor as Weatherman: Medical Topography in Nineteenth-Century New Jersey," *Journal of the Rutgers University Libraries* 62, (2006): 59-74, http://jrul.libraries.rutgers.edu (accessed July 2, 2010).

of medical practice in Beverly, praised the pure water, paucity of mosquitoes, and lack of "miasmatic influences." "Invalids resorting to this place," wrote Townsend, "have almost invariably been restored to health, or gone away benefited, their cases having become more amenable to treatment through the influence of the climate." In particular, those with "rheumatic complaints" were often able to dispense with medications in the healthful milieu of Beverly.[23] Whether permanent residents or seasonal visitors, health-seekers and the worried well were, after all, important clients of the medical profession.

In 1871, in his capacity as a municipal elected office-holder or appointee, he proposed to the Beverly governing board that a Civil War monument be erected at the "National Cemetery at this place." Perhaps memories of his father's service at Beverly's Civil War hospital and his own service at Gettysburg inspired this patriotic gesture. Townsend himself served on a second committee (the first having made no progress) formed in 1872; the committee requested and received ten thousand dollars from the state government for the erection of the memorial. Committee members visited Civil War monuments at Gettysburg, Washington, and other cities before making their recommendations. The monument, carved in Italy, was unveiled in 1875.[24]

Townsend, of course, identified himself primarily as a physician, whatever the extent of his community service. Many physicians of the day participated in political activities and contributed in one way or another to social welfare. In general, individual physicians identified strongly with their town or region. Their day-to-day medical horizons were local. Medical practice, including surgery, was largely domestic. Middle and upper class patients were routinely seen and treated in their homes. American

---

[23] Townsend, *Suburban Homes*, 5-6. "Miasmatic influences" referred to disease-causing emanations from putrefying organic matter in the soil; prior to the acceptance of the germ theory, many epidemic diseases and fevers (such as malaria) were believed to have their origins in miasmas. Townsend's medical comments are reproduced in Wade, "Historic Homes and Genealogy," 129-31.

[24] Stanley Yoka and Ethel Salamone, "Bits of the Past," in Paragraph Club, *Beverly: A Local History*, 263-66.

hospitals in the decades after the Civil War mainly served the poor and destitute, although most of these were also treated in their homes. Hospitals, often originating in urban almshouses through the charitable impulses of leading citizens, offered no advantage of skilled nursing care, medical technology, or in-house surgical or medical expertise. Burlington County opened a small hospital in Mt. Holly (the county seat, about twelve miles to the southeast of Beverly) in 1880 for charitable cases, but Townsend was not on the staff.[25] He did, however, participate in discussions about the hospital early in 1889 at a meeting of the county medical society.[26]

The practitioners in Burlington County considered themselves isolated and well out of the race for scientific prominence. A member of the Burlington County Medical Society wrote in 1866:

> As physicians, neither the past nor present generation of practitioners in Burlington County have aimed at scientific prominence. Isolated as we are, we have not the advantage of that attrition, which in compact communities burnishes the crude mineral into the polished gem, but sound practical good sense has at all times been characteristic of our physicians.[27]

From the outset of his civilian medical career, Townsend enthusiastically participated in the intellectual life of the professional community in which he found himself. At a meeting of the Burlington County Medical Society on July 12, 1864, a motion was

---

[25]   Joel R. Gardner, *Neighbor Caring for Neighbor: The History of the Medical Staff, Memorial Hospital of Burlington County, 1880-1995* (Burlington: Memorial Health Alliance, ca.1996); Burlington County Hospital Board of Managers, *Sixth Annual Report of the Board of Managers of Burlington County Hospital, Mt. Holly,* (1866), Special Collections and University Archives, Rutgers University, New Brunswick, NJ.

[26]   *Burlington County Medical Society Minute Book: 1869-1893* (entry April 13, 1880), Burlington County Medical Society Records, University of Medicine and Dentistry of New Jersey Special Collections, Newark, NJ.

[27]   [J.P. Coleman?], "Reports of District Societies, Burlington County," *TMSNJ* (1866): 150.

made by one of the nine members present to invite the newcomer to "take part in the discussions and partake of dinner with the society." Townsend jumped right in with a report on a case of uterine disease. At the next meeting in October, 1864, he was elected to membership by unanimous vote of sixteen assembled members. Perhaps recognizing his energy and enthusiasm (and their own small numbers), the members elected him vice president in January, 1865. In January, 1866, less than two years after arriving in Beverly, Townsend was elected president of the Burlington County Medical Society.[28] He was chosen as a delegate to the annual meeting of the Medical Society of New Jersey in 1866.[29] A year later, he was secretary of the county society, charged with conveying annual reports on the health of the county and the activities of member physicians to the state society.[30] He continued in this post until 1877, noting that he had not missed a single meeting in nine years.[31]

The tally of Burlington County Medical Society members in 1866 was eighteen, with an additional nineteen regular physicians who practiced in the county but who were not members of the county society.[32] Attendance at meetings, held quarterly in Mount Holly at Bodine's Hotel in the 1860s and at the Regan Hotel in the early 1870s, was necessarily limited by the expanse and rural nature of Burlington County; typically, eight to twelve members were present at meetings in the 1860s. In the late 1870s, meetings alternated between Burlington (City) and Mt. Holly.[33] There were also eight or nine homeopaths in Burlington County (not members of the county or state medical societies), most of whom were "professedly homeopathic, but practically eclectic" in their

---

[28]   *Secretary's Book: Burlington County Medical Society: 1829-1868* (entry January 9, 1866).
[29]   "Members of District Medical Societies: Burlington County," *TMSNJ* (1868): 6; "Delegates," *TMSNJ* (1866): 4.
[30]   "List of Members of District Societies," *TMSNJ* (1867): 279.
[31]   *Burlington County Medical Society Minute Book: 1869-1893* (entry October 9, 1877).
[32]   "Regular Physicians in New Jersey: 1866," *TMSNJ* (1866): 313.
[33]   *Burlington County Medical Society Minute Book: 1869-1893* (entry July 8, 1877).

professional approach to patients, suggesting that they practiced both regular and homeopathic medicine.[34]

Addison W. Taylor, M.D., who had served a medical apprenticeship with a Princeton physician and received his medical degree in 1871 from the University of Pennsylvania, opened a practice in Beverly in 1872, by which time Townsend had been for some years the sole physician in town. To complement and supplement his medical practice, Taylor was proprietor of the pharmacy in Beverly.[35] He was a member of the Burlington County Medical Society from 1872 and was named secretary to succeed Townsend in 1877, a post he held for over twenty-five years.[36] It was said that the Burlington County Medical Society was "justly proud of his fine penmanship."[37] When Townsend left Beverly for Camden in 1883, Taylor was the sole member of the Burlington County Medical Society in practice in Beverly and remained so until his death from "paralysis" in 1903.[38]

Solo practice was the norm, but Townsend and Taylor called upon each other for consultation in difficult cases. In 1875, for example, Townsend reported to the county medical society that "my friend, Dr. Taylor" called upon him to assist in a case of placenta praevia (a potentially fatal obstetrical complication in which the placenta lies sufficiently low to partially or completely obstruct the birth canal, leading to hemorrhage).[39]

---

[34]   [J.P. Coleman], "Reports of District Societies: Burlington County Medical Society," *TMSNJ* (1866): 150.

[35]   *Biographical Review, Volume XIX, Containing Life Sketches of Leading Citizens of Burlington and Camden Counties, New Jersey* (Boston: Biographical Review Publishing Company, 1897), 189-90.

[36]   *Burlington County Medical Society Minute Book: 1869-1893* (entry October 9, 1877); "Members of District Medical Societies: Burlington County," *TMSNJ* (1903): 16.

[37]   *Biographical Review*, 190.

[38]   Taylor's correct date of death (21 February 1903) is documented in his obituary, "Addison W. Taylor," *Journal of the Medical Society of New Jersey* 1 (1904-1905): 161; incorrect date of death (1904) from American Medical Association, *Directory of Deceased American Physicians* (Chicago: American Medical Association, 1993), 1526.

[39]   S.C. Thornton, "Reports of District Societies: Burlington County," *TMSNJ* (1875): 115.

Autopsies, when permission could be obtained from the family, affirmed the self-identity of the physician as a medical scientist in the tradition of French empiricism and later German laboratory medicine. Autopsies were an important form of medical education and were usually conducted by the attending physician with the assistance of professional colleagues. From a practical point of view, the autopsy provided conclusive evidence (by contemporary standards) of the physician's correct management of the case; the presence of other physicians was critical, lest the treating physician be accused of burying his mistakes. In 1875, for example, Townsend was assisted by Taylor in conducting an autopsy in a complicated case involving the post-partum death of a woman who had been under his care for over a decade.[40] In the same year, Dr. S.C. Thornton of Moorestown, Burlington County, asked Townsend and a second physician (not a member of the county medical society) to conduct an autopsy on a teenager who had died of peritonitis.[41] This suggests that Townsend was considered by his colleagues to be a scientific physician and a man whose opinion was reliable.

New Jersey's county medical societies reported to the venerable Medical Society of New Jersey (formed in 1766), which in turn fell under the umbrella of the American Medical Association as that organization gained strength in the latter half of the nineteenth century. (The Medical Society of New Jersey had sent ten delegates from across the state to the first meeting of the national organization in Philadelphia in 1847.)[42] Membership in the county society was limited to physicians with an M.D. degree from a recognized medical school; in some cases, applicants submitted themselves for oral examination by a committee of the county society. "Irregular" physicians, including homeopathic and eclectic practitioners, were not recognized by the county

---

[40]   EPT, "Case of Chronic Splenitis," *TMSNJ* (1875): 118.
[41]   S.C. Thornton, "Reports of District Societies: Burlington County," *TMSNJ* (1875): 114.
[42]   Fred B. Rogers and A. Reasoner Sayre, *The Healing Art: A History of the Medical Society of New Jersey, 1766-1966* (Trenton, NJ: Medical Society of New Jersey, 1966), 94.

and state medical societies and were denied membership during Townsend's years in Burlington County.

Until 1890, there was no effective state medical licensing law in New Jersey; membership in the county and state societies was a *de facto* "seal of approval" from the regular medical profession. Prior to 1890, registration rather than state licensing was the only legal requirement for medical practice in New Jersey. Registration consisted of filing a "careful Latin copy" of a medical school diploma (from virtually any medical school) with the county clerk's office in Mt. Holly, together with payment of a small fee.[43]

By 1880, thirty-five regular physicians were registered in Burlington County. All but a few were graduates of the University of Pennsylvania or Jefferson Medical School, both in Philadelphia. In addition, there were seven homeopaths, one veterinarian (an 1872 graduate of the New Jersey School of Veterinary Surgery in Trenton), and three practitioners of "doubtful" credentials (two from the Eclectic Medical College of Philadelphia and one from the Philadelphia University of Medicine and Surgery).[44]

As an active member of the Burlington County Medical Society, Townsend contributed to educational activities and to the county reports forwarded annually to the Medical Society of New Jersey. In 1866, shortly after arriving in Beverly, he described the case of an infant who was cured of chills by injections (referring to rectal "injections" by enema) of quinine and prepared a report on the treatment of *cholera morbus* (an obsolete term for non-specific gastroenteritis, not to be confused with epidemic cholera). In the course of the year, Townsend also described an unusual case of constipation caused by bile stones in the intestine; he showed the bile stones, passed in the stools, to his colleagues at the county medical society meeting. He also reported the case of an elderly

---

[43]   For a historical overview of medical registration and licensing in New Jersey, see David L. Cowen, *Medicine and Health in New Jersey: A History* (Princeton: D. Van Nostrand, 1964), 69-71.

[44]   "List of Physicians," *CP* 2, no. 3 (August 1881): 79-80. *TMSNJ* gave a slightly different count for 1880, listing twenty-seven regular physicians; not all registered physicians were members of the county or state medical societies. "Members of the District Medical Societies: Burlington County," *TMSNJ* (1880): 6.

man with gangrene of the toe. The patient had left Townsend's practice to consult a sectarian practitioner. When Townsend was called back in to see the case, he found that the man had consulted "not only all the old ladies of the neighborhood, but the Homeopathic, African, and other irregulars within reach." The infection had spread to the lower leg, but the patient eventually recovered under Townsend's care.[45]

Townsend's most valuable contribution to the county medical society was a tabulation of his medical activities during the year 1868. A colleague commented that Townsend's table "exhibited at a glance the innumerable modifications of disease occurring in changeable climates, where no devastating epidemics annually scourge the land."[46] In the course of 1868, his third or fourth year in practice, Townsend saw 349 cases with fourteen deaths. Seventy-one of the cases were "autumnal fevers," and forty were obstetrical. A simple calculation will show that Townsend saw, on the average, one case per day. Although some cases involved hours and sometimes days of bedside attendance, he clearly was neither well remunerated nor overly busy with his practice.[47]

All regular physicians of the period were sorely vexed by competitors who lacked the imprimatur of a diploma from a legitimate medical school. Townsend did not hesitate to join the attack on the "irregulars." The "African" physician mentioned in Townsend's gangrene case was no doubt James Still, remembered today as the "black doctor of the Pines," a self-educated herbalist from Medford, Burlington County and a constant thorn in the side of the regular practitioners.[48] The son of former slaves and brother of the well-known Philadelphia abolitionist William Still, James Still had been raised in poverty in the New Jersey Pine Barrens. The resentment of the regular physicians was based not only on the racial prejudices of the day, but also on the fact that Still was thriving financially and enjoyed a good regional reputation

---

[45]   EPT, "Special Cases by Dr. E.P. Townsend," *TMSNJ* (1866): 159.
[46]   J.P. Coleman, "Reports of District Societies: Burlington County," *TMSNJ* (1869): 115-16.
[47]   EPT, "Tabular Statement of Diseases," 126.
[48]   Sandra W. Moss, "James Still and the Regulars: The Struggle for Legitimacy," *New Jersey Medicine* 98 (October 2001): 39-44.

among white residents. In 1866, one of Townsend's colleagues from Burlington County described Still as an "Ethiopian enjoying a large and lucrative practice."[49]

County proceedings, including papers and reports of cases, were routinely submitted to the state society for publication in the *Transactions of the Medical Society of New Jersey*. In 1873 Townsend submitted his report of a case of criminal abortion in which he was obliged to surgically intervene to prevent death from sepsis. Using a probe fashioned from a male catheter, he was able to open an obstruction in the cervical os (lower portion of the uterus that dilates during labor and delivery), allowing drainage of "an intensely fetid discharge." He reminded his readers that this was "one more testimony against the criminal abortionists plying their infernal trade . . . ." Though he did not say so, he was undoubtedly pleased that he had successfully improvised by fashioning an instrument to save his patient's life. Country practitioners were often forced to rely on Yankee ingenuity, and it was something of a source of pride for Townsend that country physicians had the edge on urban practitioners in applying such skills. Some years later, on the first page of the first issue of the *Country Practitioner*, he praised the "good common sense" of the country doctor, "making his syringes in emergencies from hogs' bladders, and filing nozzles for them out of thigh bones of chickens, making surgical splints out of old shingles with his jack knife . . . ."[50]

Townsend's 1873 report to the Medical Society of New Jersey featured several cases of rheumatism and gout in which he had used "propylamin. chlorid." [sic], a drug which his father had favored in his Pennsylvania practice.[51] He was undoubtedly gratified to note that one of his patients had failed to find relief at the hands of "the best surgeons of London, Paris, Rome, and Venice" before coming to Beverly.[52] The drug continued to serve

[49] [J.P. Coleman], "Reports of District Societies: Burlington County," *TMSNJ* (1866): 150.

[50] [EPT], "To Medical Practitioners," *CP* 1, no. 1 (June, 1879): 1.

[51] W.W. Townsend, "Propylamine Chloride in Acute Inflammatory Rheumatism," *CP* 1, no. 5 (October 1879): 147-49.

[52] EPT, "Cases by Dr. Townsend," *TMSNJ* (1873): 136.

Townsend well in 1875, when he successfully treated unusually severe cases of "inflammatory rheumatism."[53] In 1869, he reported to the society on his experience with hypodermic medication. The use of hypodermic syringes was still experimental in American practice, suggesting that Townsend was eager to embrace new technologies.[54] A lifelong enthusiasm for veratrum viride (an arterial relaxant derived from green hellebore) was evident by 1873. Townsend told his Burlington County colleagues that in cases of pneumonia, veratrum viride, "proved itself absolutely master of the situation in the first stage of the disease."[55]

On at least one occasion, Townsend took on the role of preceptor to a young medical student. In October, 1880, he informed his colleagues in the county society that "in accordance with an act of the State Society, he desired to present a young man for examination preliminary to his entering upon the Study of Medicine . . . . The committee reported favorably as to the qualification of Mr. [illegible, crossed out] Alfred Porter, Dr. Townsend's student."[56] By the 1880s, medical apprenticeship with an established physician was one component of a proper American medical education—the other component was a two-year attendance at a medical school. Nothing else is known of Townsend's prospective apprentice or of the success of the preceptorship.

The isolation of small town practice was nowhere more evident than in the reports of physicians forced to cope with the most terrifying malady of pregnancy, puerperal convulsions (eclampsia or toxemia in modern terms).[57] Townsend faced one

53   S.C. Thornton, "Reports of District Societies: Burlington County, *TMSNJ* (1875): 115-16.
54   J.P. Coleman, "Reports of District Societies: Burlington County," *TMSNJ* (1869): 115. For a history of hypodermic administration of medications, see Norman Howard-Jones, "A Critical Study of the Origins and Early Development of Hypodermic Medication," *Journal of the History of Medicine and the Allied Sciences* 2 (1947): 201-48.
55   S.C. Thornton, "Reports of District Societies: Burlington County," *TMSNJ* (1873): 134.
56   *Burlington County Medical Society Minute Book: 1869-1893* (entry October 3, 1880).
57   Sandra W. Moss, "The Power to Terrify: Eclampsia in Nineteenth-Century American Practice," *Journal of Obstetrical, and Gynecologic, and Neonatal Nursing* 31 (2002): 514-20; Sandra W. Moss, "The Most Dreaded Complication of Labor: The Early

such case in 1871. The patient was a nineteen-year-old girl with convulsions occurring every fifteen minutes. To save the mother, he extracted the fetus after crushing the skull, a procedure called cranioclasty. In the decades before hospital-based Caesarian deliveries became practical in American, cranioclasty allowed the physician to extract the fetal head and body parts piecemeal in order to terminate the pregnancy and save the life of the mother; this was applied both to *in utero* fetal deaths and undeliverable live fetuses. Despite his best efforts, Townsend was helpless to prevent the death of the mother some twenty hours later.[58]

In 1873, he once again saw a woman through labor complicated by puerperal convulsions, "the most horrible condition that both patient and accoucheur [obstetrical attendant] can be placed in." Veratrum viride, Townsend's favored drug in medical emergencies, saved the day. Townsend understood veratrum, an arterial relaxant administered by "endermic" (i.e. subcutaneous) injection, to relieve excessive blood flow to the brain and promote relaxation of the cervix.[59] Years later, in the *Country Practitioner*, Townsend described another case of eclampsia with preservation of the life of the mother: "What physician that has stood by the bedside of a patient, writhing with puerperal convulsions, surrounded by frightened friends and attendants, does not shudder, as his memory dwells upon it."[60] For the country doctor, alone except for anguished family, neighbors, and perhaps a midwife, the care of a parturient who was convulsing (and, mercifully, unconscious or semi-conscious for hours on end), was truly terrifying. The welfare of the infant could be only of secondary concern to a doctor faced with the imminent death of the mother in the decades before Caesarian section and the myriad other tools of twentieth-century obstetrics.

Treatment of Eclampsia in New Jersey," *New Jersey Medicine* 98 (April 2001): 43-48.

[58]   S.C. Thornton, "Reports of District Societies: Burlington County," *TMSNJ* (1871): 256-57.

[59]   EPT, "Cases by Dr. Townsend: Obstetrics," *TMSNJ* (1873): 137.

[60]   EPT, "Puerperal Eclampsia, *CP* 1, no. 2 (July 1879): 26, no terminal question mark in the original.

All obstetric cases with poor outcomes seemed to weigh heavily on Townsend. From 1864 to 1875, he attended a woman with a stenotic (narrowed) uterine canal and recurrent abdominal pain. Townsend surgically widened the canal, and the woman subsequently became pregnant. The pregnancy was complicated by hyperemesis gravidarum (severe vomiting of pregnancy), whereupon Townsend substituted rectal "injections" (enemas delivered rectally by a large syringe) of beef tea for the oral diet she could not tolerate. A difficult labor with a forceps delivery was complicated by hemorrhage from an atonic uterus (failure of the uterus to contract after expulsion of the infant). Townsend administered the drug ergot to induce uterine contractions and applied external pressure over the lower abdomen to force the uterus to contract. To hasten constriction of bleeding vessels, he applied cold in the form of snowballs introduced into the vagina![61] The patient died about a week after delivery, having suffered recurring abdominal pain, most notably pain in the left upper quadrant of the abdomen over the area of the spleen. "The privilege of post mortem examination having been solicited and granted," Townsend and his local colleague found to their surprise that the liver was grossly enlarged and the spleen dark in color with signs of softening and inflammation. He concluded that the splenic disease ("splenitis") had contributed to her death from "debility" by destroying her red blood cells and, furthermore, had been responsible for her many years of abdominal pain.

Once again, Townsend reflected unhappily on the emotional burdens of the physician faced with such a case: "I am aware that in my hurried description of the this case, I have failed to convey any idea of the difficulties I have experienced in managing it; not only in former years, but during her last sickness . . . . I am inclined to cry out that money is no sufficient remuneration for the assumption of such responsibilities."[62]

In 1876, Townsend was invited to be one of two "essayists" for the annual meeting of the Medical Society of New Jersey to be held in Cape May. The second essayist was Dr. R.M. Bateman

---

61   EPT, "Case of Chronic Splenitis,"119.
62   Ibid., 118-19.

of Cumberland County, also in the southern part of the state. Bateman's essay, when published in the *Transactions of the Medical Society of New Jersey*, ran to some twenty pages. His topic was "Mental Pathology and Criminal Law."[63] Never one to tolerate tedious meetings or long-winded speakers, Townsend conscientiously crafted a six-page essay entitled "Medical Heroism." An announcement from the chair to the effect that time constraints demanded that the two essays be read out by title only and referred to the committee on publication, must have been a harsh blow indeed.[64] Whether Townsend was furious or merely irritated must be left to the imagination.

In his essay, Townsend listed the accepted moral virtues of the good physician: integrity, purity, sympathy for suffering, and charity. To these he added bravery and heroism. The bravery of which Townsend wrote referred to the courage to lay aside medical school lectures, reference works, and clinical training in the face of clinical uncertainty. Patients differed in their circumstances and constitutions, making it necessary, in some cases, to depart from "plans of treatment that dare to be taken as an infallible guide." The attending physician must

> . . . cut himself loose from their thralldom and pursue such a course as his own judgment may dictate, even though adverse to the recognized practice, with a full knowledge that if he does so, and the case terminate unfavorably, he will be open to criticism and censure.[65]

A general physician would inevitably be forced to make hard choices not only in obstetrical practice, but in other therapeutic dilemmas such as the treatment of children with life-threatening illness. For example, in the all-too-frequent case of a child suffocating from throat obstruction secondary to "membranous croup" (diphtheria) the physician had to decide quickly between "meekly" ordering the usual gentle remedies or heroically treating

---

63   R.M. Bateman, "Mental Pathology and Criminal Law," *TMSNJ* (1876): 77-95.

64   EPT, "Medical Heroism" 96-101; William Pierson, "Minutes: One Hundred and Tenth Annual Meeting, Medical Society of New Jersey," *TMSNJ* (1876): 26.

65   EPT, "Medical Heroism," 99.

boldly with veratrum and emetics. The consequences to the physician, should the patient die, lay not in malpractice litigation, but in loss of reputation. Townsend ended with an exhortation to his readers to find the courage to depart from standard teachings and theories when the situation calls for it—it is what the patient and family have a right to expect:

> He who takes no step, except at the instigation of his medical authorities, and prescribes after their recommendations only, soon becomes a mere routinist, and in those acute cases where death stares the patient squarely in the face, too often finds that while he is weaving theories, his patient has slipped from his fingers, for want of prompt assistance.[66]

Having stated his case and assured his audience that he was no doubt preaching to a choir of physicians who were of a similar mind, Townsend closed by citing the merit of brevity in a medical essay. Townsend's life as a country practitioner was anything but dull. He seemed to be one of those physicians who saw instructive value in each case and had the satisfaction of seeing a number of his reports in print, even before he founded his own journal. But nothing in Beverly quite matched the excitement and misery of medical practice deep in the Amazon on the border of Bolivia!

---

[66]   Ibid., 100-1.

CHAPTER 4

THE NEWS FROM BRAZIL:
ADVENTURES IN THE AMAZON

At an October 9th, 1877, meeting of the Burlington County Medical Society, Townsend announced that he was resigning as secretary and anticipated a three-year absence from the state. A colleague "expressed the regret of the Society at the departure of Dr. Townsend from among us after so many years of pleasant and profitable association and moved that he be elected an honorary member . . . . Dr. Thornton wished Dr. Townsend a safe passage and hoped that he might be well delivered."[1]

The good wishes of his colleagues for a safe passage were appropriate. For reasons that are not clear, Townsend signed up as a physician (one of at least three) on a railroad-building expedition in the deep interior of South America. Named for one of the organizing engineers, the Collins expedition sought to build a railroad around unnavigable portions of the Madeira River, a major Amazon tributary, on the Brazilian-Bolivian border. The ultimate rationale for the project was the potential linkage of American commercial interests to the interior of South America. As time went on, the practical goal of surviving members of the

---

[1]   *Burlington County Medical Society Minute Book: 1869-1893* (entry October 9, 1877), Burlington County Medical Society Records, University of Medicine and Dentistry of New Jersey Special Collections, Newark, NJ.

expedition, both laborers and managers, was to return home alive.[2]

The *Beverly Weekly Visitor* for November 10, 1877 carried notices to the effect that Dr. Townsend was offering for sale a "good family horse, a new sleigh, buffalo robe, blanket, and food chest . . . and a new set of carriage harness." He would "dispose of the above goods at a low figure, if applied for soon." Beverly residents, continued the notice, were losing a "physician of skill and experience," while gaining a man with "glowing recommendations from the citizens of Burlington."[3] H.M. Harvey, M.D., had already moved from the nearby city of Burlington to Beverly and taken over Townsend's practice. Harvey's tenure in Burlington prior to moving to Beverly must have been brief, since he was first elected to the Burlington County Medical Society in April, 1876.[4] He did indeed take over Townsend's practice, posting his "business card" with the phrase "successor to Dr. Townsend" in the *Beverly Weekly Visitor*. This notice ran from November 24, 1877, through at least mid-1878.

How did Townsend learn about the Brazil venture? A Philadelphia merchant, Hugh Hamilton, a "townsman from Beverly," was involved in negotiating the contracts for the expedition.[5] Other residents of Beverly also signed up. One citizen of Beverly predicted that no one who joined the expedition would return alive; not only was the construction concern's steamship (the

[2] Unless otherwise noted, information about the Collins expedition is from Neville B. Craig, *Recollections of an Ill-Fated Expedition to the Headwaters of the Madeira River in Brazil* (Philadelphia: J.B. Lippincott, 1907). Page references are given for comments relevant to Townsend and the medical aspects of the expedition. The full text is available on-line at http://books.google.com/books, enter "Recollections of an Ill-Fated Voyage."

[3] "Local Matters," *Beverly Weekly Visitor*, November 10, 1877. *Beverly Weekly Visitor*, a four-page weekly preserved on microfilm at Rutgers University, has gaps from August, 1878, through January, 1879. No copies beyond early 1879 could be located.

[4] *Burlington County Medical Society Minute Book: 1869-1893* (entry April 11, 1876).

[5] Craig, *Recollections*, 67-69; "Local Items," *Beverly Weekly Visitor*, November 10, 1878.

Mercedita), an "old tub," but "the Miasma or some other fatal disease" would quickly kill off the adventurers.[6]

Townsend's long-term plans are unknown. Perhaps he anticipated substantial remuneration, either from salary or a share in the profits, sufficient to support his family for some years. He may have contemplated a change in location after his return from South America, having taken the major step of selling his practice before departing. In any case, a trip of three years to the interior of the Amazon seemed like a risky venture for a young physician with a dependent wife and children! Townsend's family remained behind in Beverly, as very few wives accompanied the expedition.[7]

Over two hundred American personnel, among them Townsend, sailed from Philadelphia on January 2, 1878, aboard the *Mercedita*. It is not clear whether Townsend was chief physician once in Brazil, but he was named in the newspapers as being "in charge of medical operations" at the time of the *Mercedita's* departure.[8] A letter to the local newspaper from a Beverly resident aboard the *Mercedita*, in commenting on the uncomfortable voyage, included news of Townsend: "Our leading man aboard is the Doctor as he is here and there wherever he is called upon, ready to do duty since he has found his 'sea legs.'" The writer, signed "Hard Tack," mentioned the Beverly men in particular: "All our Beverlonians send their respects though your paper, to friends to whom they were not able to write. It is quite laughable to see the Doctor receive his patients." Various "Beverlonians" were assisting on the vessel as volunteer policemen, mess captains, and cooks' mates.[9]

A two-month voyage by way of Barbados, Pará (in northeastern Brazil at the mouth of the Amazon), and the Amazon and Madeira Rivers brought the expedition to the falls near San

---

6   "Local Items," *Beverly Weekly Visitor*, January 5, 1878.

7   Among the few accompanying wives was a Mrs. Packer, who was from Beverly; "Hard Tack" (pen name), "Life on Board the *Mercedita*," *Beverly Weekly Visitor*, February 16, 1878.

8   "Expedition to Brazil," *New York Times*, January 3, 1878.

9   "Hard Tack," "Life on Board the *Mercedita*," *Beverly Weekly Visitor*, February 16, 1878.

Antonio, close to the Bolivian border. Previously abandoned by British adventurers, San Antonio was a pestilential outpost with no amenities. It would serve as expedition headquarters and the center of medical operations. A second ship, the *Metropolis*, bound from Philadelphia with men and supplies for the expedition was wrecked in late January, 1878, off the North Carolina coast. By the time vessels bearing further personnel, equipment, and medical supplies arrived in San Antonio in June, 1878, the crude settlement was short of food and vital medications such as quinine. Each day saw another death due to disease and debility.[10]

At least three physicians were working at San Antonio by mid-year, but Townsend was probably the first on the scene, having arrived with the *Mercedita* in early March. Most laborers were either Irish-Americans or Italian-Americans recruited in the Philadelphia area; the Italians were considered troublemakers by the expedition leaders. Additional local Indian laborers were also hired as the project progressed. A guard shot and wounded in an altercation with a mutinous Italian laborer provided the first surgical challenge for the expedition's physicians. Issuing frequent progress bulletins, the physicians, (dubbed "the mighty triumvirate" by the historian of the expedition), became, for a few hours, the center of attention at San Antonio. The wounded guard had, as it turned out, suffered only a minor flesh wound and was treated with whiskey by the "disgusted disciples of Aesculapius."[11]

Almost all expedition members, including those in San Antonio and others working in peripheral work encampments or in surveying parties, suffered from malaria, dysentery and other diseases endemic to the region; scurvy was also diagnosed as food supplies became inadequate.[12] Interestingly, the book-length account, *Recollections of an Ill-Fated Expedition to the Headwaters of the Madeira River in Brazil*, written years later by Neville B. Craig, an expedition member, did not mention any cases of yellow fever during the months in the deep Amazon, although

---

[10] Craig, *Recollections*, 219.

[11] Ibid., 230-2.

[12] Ibid., 239.

some unfortunate Americans did fall ill with yellow fever while awaiting passage home from the eastern port city of Pará.[13]

By June, 1878, a mere three months after their arrival at the deep Amazon base, invalids from the chief engineer down to workmen were being sent home by the medical officers, who continued to struggle with a shortage of quinine and other medications.[14] The physicians resorted to buying quinine from expedition members who had had the foresight to stockpile personal supplies of the drug before leaving the United States. The doctors also began cutting their dwindling supply of quinine with sugar to keep confidence and spirits up. It is unlikely that the physicians themselves escaped attacks of fever, whether from contaminated drinking water or infected mosquitoes.

A primitive hospital was soon overflowing with fever cases. The hospital orderly, an officious and slovenly character with no medical training, doubled as nurse and gravedigger. Most of the men in peripheral jungle encampments simply cared for themselves with quinine (if available) or confinement to their hammocks. In late June, Townsend announced that close to two hundred men at San Antonio were unfit for further service in the Amazonian climate. Well over half the men in the region of San Antonio were on the sick list.[15]

The graveyard at San Antonio was dubbed "the banana patch," and it was too quickly occupied. July and August of 1878 were particularly unhealthy. Commander Thomas Oliver Selfridge, a visiting American naval officer on a surveying mission to the Amazon, declared that he had never in his life "seen a more unhappy and unhealthy body of men than the workmen on the railroad."[16] Some expedition members died in outlying encampments and on various surveying and engineering missions to the proposed train route. Many invalided and discharged laborers had not been paid and had no financial resources for the trip back to the United States. Of these, an unknown number died in makeshift small craft heading back down the Amazon to Pará. Some of

---

[13]   Ibid., 402.
[14]   Ibid., 268-300.
[15]   Ibid., 301-4.
[16]   Ibid., 383.

those who survived the trip to Pará remained destitute in that city for weeks or months. By September or October, a majority of engineers and laborers had left for home or died, although the expedition leaders carried on. An expedition physician named Whitaker, making his way back to the United States in December, arranged for some American invalids to be hospitalized at Pará, despite the fact that he found the municipal hospital to be "worse than hell."[17] Perhaps he judged the men too ill to withstand the voyage and concluded that the hospital, appalling as it was, was their best hope.

The expedition was abandoned officially in mid-1879, having foundered on problems of provisioning and contracting, manpower shortages due to disease, labor strife, financial woes, hostile terrain, aggressive fauna, miasmic climate, and general disillusionment at all levels. Certainly, disease and malnutrition played major roles in sabotaging the project. The total number of deaths among native laborers, Italian contract workers, and American expedition members is unknown. Others may have been left chronic invalids or died after returning to the United States. One estimate is that of the 941 employees who set out from the United States, some 222 were known to have died, for a mortality rate of over twenty-three percent.[18]

It is not known exactly when Townsend returned to Beverly or the state of his health when he arrived. He had planned a to be away for three years, but appears to have left for home after about a year. Either Townsend was too ill to continue as a physician to the expedition or his services became superfluous when conditions became intolerable and the expedition failed. Unfortunately, local Beverly newspapers from the last half of 1878 have not survived, but a January, 1879, issue of the *Beverly Weekly Visitor* carried a notice of Townsend's regular office hours. Townsend seems to have resumed his old practice, as Dr. Harvey's name disappeared from the Beverly newspaper by 1879.[19] Minutes from late 1878 are missing from the secretary's book of the Burlington County Medical Society, but Townsend was present at the January 1879

---

[17] Ibid., 400.
[18] Ibid., 425.
[19] "Business Cards," *Beverly Weekly Visitor*, January 2, 1879.

meeting, as was Harvey. Apparently there was some friction between the two men in late 1878, probably related to Townsend's earlier-than-expected return and his desire to resume his practice. Dr. Taylor, recording secretary and a Beverly colleague of both men, reported in the January 1879 minutes:

> The report of the Censors on Dr. Harvey's charge against Dr. Townsend was received and after some discussion adopted . . . . Dr. Townsend made some remarks to the effect that he regretted the trouble between himself and Dr. Harvey had occurred before the society and that he wished to be reinstated in his former record: these views were adopted as the feelings of the society.[20]

A year later, upon founding his journal, the *Country Practitioner*, Townsend published some brief observations of Brazilian health and medical practice in the first issue. While in Brazil, he had communicated with local physicians, visited hospitals (" . . . for that country very fair specimens of cleanliness and comfort, [but] in this country they would not be tolerated."), and observed diseases among the indigenous peoples. Townsend described his trip up the Amazon and Madeira Rivers, closely observing the folk medicine practices of indigenous Bolivians. He was intrigued by the typical medical "kit" of indigenous river travelers, which included jaborandi (to stimulate perspiration and respiratory secretions), coca (a nerve stimulant and tonic, the precursor of cocaine), extract of guarana (caffeine, used in "cephalic" or brain fevers), and quinae (unrefined quinine, of great value in "periodic fevers" due to malaria.)[21]

Following his return from Brazil to Beverly, Townsend "made considerable use of Jaborandi and erythroxylin coca, with favorable results." He also had some success with guarana for facial neuralgias. In the nineteenth century, drug trials were almost always conducted by individual practitioners. By modern standards, such trials were unregulated and lacked standardization.

---

[20]   *Burlington County Medical Society Minute Book: 1869-1893* (entry January 14, 1879).

[21]   EPT, "Medical Practice in Brazil," *CP* 2, no. 3 (August 1880): 75-76.

Informed consent and the other machinery of modern clinical testing were unknown. Nevertheless, these anecdotal drug trials represented the medical science of the day. Experience with new or unfamiliar medications was often reported to medical journals; conclusions were based on empirical observations rather than statistics. Aware that his limited observations were inconclusive, Townsend ended his brief report on Brazilian folk medicines with a plea for comments or additional articles from his readers and added some opinions on jaborandi from the *British Medical Journal* and the *Hospital Gazette.*[22]

A second article about South America appeared a year later in the second volume of the *Country Practitioner*, and focused on "Medical Practice in Brazil." Of interest to Townsend and his readers were the measures taken by Brazil with respect to physician licensing:

> The Empire of Brazil strikes the nail on the head, by refusing all diplomas and credentials and demanding under a heavy penalty in money and imprisonment that every person before attempting to practice in her domains shall pass a rigid examination in the Portuguese language before a medical board at Bahaia.[23]

New Jersey physicians had long sought legislation to regulate the practice of medicine and "prevent imposters from assuming the functions of physicians." Despite the strict licensing laws in Brazil, Townsend found the level of practice there very low, physician night calls non-existent, and hospital standards of cleanliness unacceptable. The generally poor health of Brazilian Indians—"poor devils with their ulcerated legs and toeless feet"—led Townsend to conclude that native remedies were "over-extolled" (among

---

[22]   [EPT], "New Remedies," *CP* 1, no. 1 (June 1879): 33. The *Hospital Gazette* probably referred to *Hospital Gazette: A Monthly Journal of Medicine and Surgery*, published from 1877 in New York. Townsend's reference to the *British Medical Journal* demonstrated his interest in keeping up to date with European, as well as American, medical progress.

[23]   EPT, "Medical Practice in Brazil," 75.

Americans), and that notwithstanding protective licensing laws, "medical intelligence was at a low ebb in the Brazils."[24]

Townsend left no known personal record of the Brazil expedition except for the two brief items in the *Country Practitioner.* Whatever his original plans had been, he resumed practice in Beverly and set out upon the new adventure of founding a medical journal.

[24]   Ibid., 77.

CHAPTER 5

THE COUNTRY PRACTITIONER LAUNCHES THE COUNTRY PRACTITIONER

John Shaw Billings, the foremost expert on medical journalism, was perhaps somewhat jaded from listing scores of failed medical journals in his review of the American medical literature. He quipped in 1879: "It is as useless to advise a man not to start a new journal as it is to advise him not to commit suicide."[1] With time on his hands and a lively intellectual curiosity, Townsend entered upon just such an enterprise in that selfsame year of 1879. He founded *The Country Practitioner; Or New Jersey Journal of Medical & Surgical Practice*, a publication that reflected his interests and filled a void in the literature of American medicine. Townsend was sole owner, editor, business and circulation manager and, very often, contributor.

The journal was a pamphlet with a sewn binding, eight and one half by six inches in size. The cover, printed on grayish-green paper, bore the title of the journal, the name of the editor, and the price ("$2.50 per annum, 25 cents single number"). Townsend sent out "specimen numbers" (free copies) of the first issue to every regular physician in the state, or, more likely, every member of the county medical societies.[2] Between issues five and six of

---

[1]   J[ohn] S[haw] Billings, "The Medical Journals of the United States," *Boston Medical and Surgical Journal* 100 (1879): 2.

[2]   [EPT] "Editorial," *CP* 1, no. 3 (August 1879): 106.

the first volume, the price dropped to $2.00 per annum. Some revenue came in from advertising (a full page for one year was $100) and there were several regular advertisers.[3]

The printer was the local Banner Steam-Power Print of Beverly. Five to ten articles in each issue included invited and submitted reports and commentaries, extracts and reprints of articles borrowed from other publications, and regular features such as "Notes on Country Practice." The articles were followed by short editorials, unsigned though clearly written by Townsend using the editorial "we," and a section of book reviews. Each issue was about forty pages long, with unpaginated advertisements on the inside front cover and at the back of the journal.

Townsend saw his potential national readership as large and geographically diverse—the base of the pyramid of American medicine. In the third issue, he wrote: "Our columns are at the disposal of County Societies and physicians from Maine to Texas, and from the Atlantic to the Pacific."[4] The first issue opened with a statement of his goals for the new journal:

> . . . to [bring] into general use the latent information possessed by every practitioner who is, and has been doing good service in his own immediate circle, fighting out of his own difficulties, when out of the reach of specialists and scientists, leaning upon his knowledge of general principles, basing his practice upon his good common sense . . . . striving and fighting his way alone through emergencies that would cause some of the great medical luminaries to stagger in their traces. Not that all country practitioners are necessarily good physicians, but that their isolation from the fraternity, and the circumstances surrounding them tend to draw out and develop—not self conceit, but self reliance, and force them to the performance of work that if it were possible they would gladly shirk by passing the case over to a specialist . . . . They see disease in its uncomplicated form more often than hospital practitioners—for their patients are among people who breathe pure country

---

3   "Advertising Rates," *CP* 1, no. 6 (November 1879): 213.
4   [EPT], "Editorial," *CP* 1, no. 3 (August 1879): 106.

air, and less often contaminated by scrofulous, syphilitic, or other constitutional taint.

Furthermore, continued Townsend, he possessed the time and skills to do the job:

> I have most seasons of the year more time than my practice demands, take great pleasure in the kind of work the management of the journal will require of me, and am not averse to turning an honest penny by the operation, if the journal lives—although I expect a doctor's luck in the latter, for many a year to come, i.e., more work than pay.

And, he warned, he would take his editor's gatekeeper duties seriously: "I shall also reserve the right to criticize any or all articles that I may accept, and hold the author of the article responsible for the defense of his views." Lest he offend his urban colleagues, he penned an added reassurance:

> In addressing country practitioners, I do not wish to discriminate in the least, or deteriorate one jot from the acknowledged ability of our city brethren . . . . [I]t is all the more their duty to be in the picket line of medical research, and send us at least some of the crumbs from the rich repasts they are enjoying.[5]

Townsend also addressed other journal editors:

> We have not originated this Journal with any hope of excelling you or filling your place, but with the hope of drawing out material which escapes you, and comes direct from the rank and file of the profession, while you send us the news from head quarters [sic].[6]

The *Country Practitioner* was launched and received a warm local reception. In winding up his 1879 history of the Burlington

---

[5]   [EPT], "To Medical Practitioners," *CP* 1, no. 1 (June 1879): 1-3.
[6]   [EPT], "To Medical Journalists," *CP* 1, no. 1 (June 1879): 35.

County Medical Society's first half century, Dr. Joseph Parrish, a practitioner in the city of Burlington and former editor of the *New Jersey Medical Reporter* (later the *New Jersey Medical and Surgical Reporter*), praised the *Country Practitioner* in a flurry of horticultural metaphors:

> One thing more it [the Burlington County Medical Society] has done; one of the last things and one of the best. Now, at the very close of our first half century, we have commenced work again in the field of journalism; not because our first effort failed [referring to Parrish's own *New Jersey Medical Reporter*], for it has not. It still bears fruit in another soil [Philadelphia], whither it was transplanted years since; but now the *Country Practitioner* begins. Its first number has just greeted us. It is a new seedling from a thriving stock. It was budded in the genial mould of this society, and is now a living fragrant plant. Its fruit time is not yet, but it will soon come, if we stand by our brother the editor and aid him in his work. Its pages should be the medium for publishing the history of Burlington County medicine for the next half century; and not an honorable name nor a worthy deed of our profession should fail of record. May the *Country Practitioner* become a power for good among us.[7]

Praise from Parrish, embodying as he did the slight history of medical journalism in New Jersey, was important to Townsend. In the first issue of the *County Practitioner*, he in turn took note of Parrish's journal: "The *Medical and Surgical Reporter,* one of the best medical journals in the country, was born in the city of Burlington, N.J., and afterward transferred by Dr. Butler, its late lamented [second] editor, to Philadelphia."[8]

---

[7] Parrish's address was reproduced in a supplement to the *Country Practitioner.* Joseph Parrish, "Historical Address," *CP* (supp.) 1, no. 2 (July 1879): 18-19. The full text of Parrish's address was also published in a pamphlet: Joseph Parrish, "Historical Address," in Burlington County Medical Society, *Semi-Centennial Anniversary of the District Medical Society for the County of Burlington,* June 17, 1879," (Banner Steam-Power Print: Beverly, NJ, 1879), 27-8.

[8] [EPT], "To Medical Practitioners," *CP* 1, no. 1 (July 1879): 2.

The *Country Practitioner* was listed in the first series of the *Index-Catalogue of the Surgeon General's Library* (1880), a definitive guide to the medical literature, both American and European. Evidently, Townsend sent a complementary copy to the library of the Surgeon General in Washington.[9] The inclusion of a complete run (twenty-seven issues) of the *Country Practitioner* in bound volumes in the library of the College of Physicians of Philadelphia and of an incomplete run of twenty-four issues at the New York Academy of Medicine suggests three possibilities: Townsend sent gratis copies to major medical libraries; the academy libraries purchased subscriptions; or members of those academies donated their copies. Today, medical school libraries in Massachusetts, Illinois, Michigan, New Orleans, and California own the *Country Practitioner*, supporting the claim that Townsend's journal had at least a small national audience.[10]

The *Country Practitioner* appeared during a period of rapid and profound transformation in American medical practice. In the last decades of the nineteenth century, the search for specific disease entities, supported ideally by clinical and laboratory research, began to compete with the older notion that diseases were due to internal imbalances and disharmonies between the patient and his environment. Physicians who saw the individual patient rather than a disease process as the proper target of therapy continued to take into account the constitution and circumstances of each patient before prescribing. For example, adherents of the older notion of disease causation might conclude that an inflamed throat in a hardy country dweller from the southern part of the country required a different therapeutic approach from that prescribed for the same inflamed throat in a pale and nervous city dweller from the north.

---

[9]   Library of the Surgeon-General's Office, *Index-Catalogue of the Library of the Surgeon-General's Office Library*, ser. 1, vol. 14 (Washington: Government Printing Office, 1880), 14:666. http://indexcat.nlm.nih.gov/ (accessed July 2, 2010). The *Index Catalogue* was largely the work of John Shaw Billings.

[10]   WorldCat Online Computer Library Center (accessed December 2, 2010)

With advances in the basic medical sciences, therapies targeted at specific identifiable and definable diseases were gradually introduced into medical practice. Historian of medicine John Harley Warner has characterized this paradigm shift as a transition from "specificity" to "universalism" in medical therapeutics. In the case of diphtheria, for example, with the application of the germ theory to the identification of the diphtheria bacterium in 1883 and the introduction of antitoxin in the 1890s, the individual patient's milieu and constitution became far less relevant—even irrelevant—to the choice of treatment.[11]

In practice, all careful physicians continued to draw on their knowledge of patients' idiosyncrasies and circumstances to guide diagnosis and therapy, even as they learned to apply laboratory and clinical science to everyday practice. In a highly competitive practice environment, in which smooth-talking charlatans and sectarians appeared to have much, and often more, to offer than "regular" physicians, it behooved men like Townsend to treat his patients as individuals and tailor therapy to their specific idiosyncrasies, perceived preferences, and expectations. A physician who "treats his patients," Townsend wrote in the *Country Practitioner* in 1879, "has a great deal better success in his profession than he who treats diseases."[12] The country doctor, seeking both to serve his unique patients and, at the same time, keep up with new medical advances coming, for the most part, from Europe, found himself with a foot in both camps. Although physicians were well aware that therapeutics had not kept pace with the spectacular advances in fields such as physiology and microbiology, conscientious country doctors wanted to offer the best scientific medical care possible, another important trump-card in their endless struggle with the sectarians and charlatans.

In his choice of articles and in his editorial comments, Townsend grappled with many of the practice issues of his day

---

[11]   John Harley Warner, "From Specificity to Universalism in Medical Therapeutics: Transformation in the 19th-Century United States," in *Sickness and Health in America: Readings in the History of Medicine and Public Health*, 3rd. ed., eds. Judith Walzer Leavitt and Ronald L. Numbers (Madison, WI: University of Wisconsin Press, 1997), 87-101.

[12]   [EPT], "City and Country Doctors," *CP* 1, no. 8 (January 1880): 261.

during the brief twenty-seven-month life of his journal. He returned often to three subjects that captured his attention: the therapeutic use of veratrum as a pharmacological substitute for bloodletting, the diagnosis and treatment of childhood diphtheria, and the life-threatening complications encountered in the minefield of obstetrical practice.

CHAPTER 6

KEEPING ABREAST: VERATRUM, DIPHTHERIA, AND OBSTETRICS

In twenty-seven monthly issues published between June 1879 and September 1881, a number of important themes emerged from the wide-ranging topics that filled each thirty-to-forty-page issue of the *Country Practitioner*. Of continuing interest to Townsend as he launched his new journal was veratrum viride (American hellebore), classified as an arterial relaxant and, as we have seen previously, favored by Townsend in obstetrical practice and the treatment of pneumonia. The use of such drugs was a refinement on the hallowed practice of phlebotomy or bloodletting. Physicians often referred to "opening a vein" or the "use of the lancet," medical shorthand for the application of a scalpel (lancet) to a superficial vein. Many of Townsend's contemporaries regretted the gradual decline of bloodletting, favored from early colonial days until the mid-nineteenth century for restoring internal balance in a wide spectrum of symptoms and diseases. Vigorous phlebotomy was employed by many New Jersey disciples of Philadelphia physician Benjamin Rush as a treatment for yellow fever in the 1790s and remained popular with some practitioners through much of the nineteenth century.[1] One New Jersey physician

---

[1] Sandra Moss, "This Destroying Scourge: Yellow Fever Epidemics of the 1790s in New Jersey," *New Jersey Heritage* 5 (2006): 10-23. Rush's "one size fits all" treatment of yellow fever also called for vigorous purging with harsh laxatives such as calomel

observed in 1863, "our lancets rust in their cases, and our former heroic remedies remain neglected on our shelves."[2] Some years later, D.E. Michener, a contributor to the *Country Practitioner* lamented: "For more than half a century I used the lancet very freely . . . And to an extent which few physicians seem willing to imitate. But now, at the age of eighty-six years, a retrospect of the past brings up vastly more regrets for the *omission* than for the *employment* of the remedy."[3]

Among the prominent late-century supporters of bloodletting was Dr. Samuel D. Gross, Townsend's former professor of surgery at Jefferson Medical College. Gross signed a letter on the subject of bloodletting to the editor of the *Country Practitioner*, "Very truly your friend":

> [I]n the course of lectures which I annually deliver in the Jefferson Medical College, I dwell with much force and emphasis upon the employment of the lancet in the early stages of inflammatory affections involving important structures, before they have been overwhelmed by inflammatory exudations. I wish to God that it were in my power to write this sentence in letters of fire upon the brain of every practicing physician and surgeon in the civilized world.[4]

Gross enclosed a copy of his address, delivered six years previously at a meeting of the American Medical Association. Townsend dutifully printed Gross' lengthy address, "A Discourse on Bloodletting Considered as a Therapeutic Agent" in the next

---

(a mercurial laxative) and jalap (a herbal laxative). Such depletive therapy, applied to patients with fever, vomiting, and diarrhea, must have hurried many victims to their deaths by adding to the dehydration and circulatory collapse caused by the underlying disease.

2 W.M. Brown, "Reports of District Societies: Essex County," *TMSNJ* (1863): 54. David L. Cowen drew my attention to this quotation in David L. Cowen, *Medicine and Health in New Jersey: A History* (Princeton: D. Van Nostrand, 1964), 33.

3 E. Michener, "Notes on Bloodletting as a Remedy," *CP* 2, no. 9 (February 1881): 289, italics in original. Michener was from Chester County, PA, and was probably known personally to Townsend.

4 Samuel D. Gross, "Correspondence," *CP* 2, no. 10 (March 1881): 331.

two issues of the *Country Practitioner*.[5] Gross was no maverick; bloodletting in pneumonia was an area of contention through much of the nineteenth century. As late as 1898, William Osler of Johns Hopkins Medical School, America's leading internist and teacher of internal medicine, supported bloodletting in severe early pneumonia in robust individuals as a means of relieving dyspnea (shortness of breath), pain and "cerebral symptoms."[6] The rationale behind bloodletting for inflammatory diseases, particularly pneumonia, was its presumed ability to reduce the signs of inflammation: "overaction of the heart, imperfect supply of nerve fluid, deranged circulation, impaired function of vital organs, and above all, from disordered structure from inflammatory deposits."[7] Because pneumonia was invariably accompanied by a rapid heartbeat, it was axiomatic that proper therapy should be directed at quieting the heart, thereby relieving the burden on the pulmonary circulation.[8]

Relying on the pulse as a guide, physicians sought to regulate the circulation with cardiac depressants such as veratrum even as bloodletting (phlebotomy) was fading from medical practice. The use of veratrum viride as an arterial relaxant was viewed by Townsend and many others as a sort of "medical phlebotomy"—a method of "quieting" the circulation temporarily without the disadvantages of bloodletting.[9]

Veratrum viride was known to slow the pulse and dilate the blood vessels. Used recklessly, it caused vascular collapse (shock) and death, a fact well known to Townsend and his contemporaries three decades before the blood pressure cuff

---

5   Samuel D. Gross "A Discourse on Bloodletting Considered as a Therapeutic Agent" *CP* 2, nos. 10, 11 (March, April 1881): 337-45, 371-78.

6   William Osler, *The Principles and Practice of Medicine*, 3rd ed. (New York: D. Appleton & Co., 1898), 135.

7   Gross, "Discourse on Bloodletting," *CP* 2, no.10, 344.

8   For a historical review of bloodletting in pneumonia, see Ralph G. DePalma, Virginia W. Hayes, and Leo R. Zacharski, "Bloodletting: Past and Present," *Journal of the American College of Surgeons* 205 (2007): 132-44.

9   Veratrum reentered the pharmacopeia some years later, being used until the 1950s to control life-threatening (malignant) hypertension and the hypertensive crisis of toxemia of pregnancy. Louis S. Goodman and Alfred Gilman, *The Pharmacological Basis of Therapeutics*, 2nd ed. (New York: Macmillan, 1955), 747-54.

was introduced into regular American practice.[10] Veratrum also caused respiratory depression, an undesirable side-effect in advanced pneumonia. But carefully monitored by a capable physician, veratrum was considered safe by those experienced in its use and convinced of its effectiveness. Wrote one New Jersey physician in 1863, " . . . cautiously administered and watched," veratrum allows the physician to "counteract at once any undue depressing action."[11]

Townsend was a strong advocate of veratrum viride in cases of inflammation and had employed it liberally since opening his practice. Applying the same rationale as the dedicated phlebotomists, he and others maintained that carefully titrated doses of veratrum calmed the circulation, thereby reducing inflammation:

> As surely as I believe that pneumonia is inflammation of the lung, and that inflammation is the result of rapid circulation of the blood—so certainly do I believe that tincture verat. viride, properly administered in the first stages [of pneumonia] will inevitably abort the disease.[12]

Like those devoted to bloodletting, Townsend believed that the rapid pulse exacerbated the engorgement of the lung. Modern physicians would conclude that such reasoning was inverted; the fast and full pulse is a physiological response to fever, infection, inflammation, and inadequate oxygenation. Therapy

---

[10]   George B. Wood, Franklin Bache, *Dispensatory of the United States of America* (Philadelphia: Lippincott, 1883), 1519-21. The blood pressure cuff, or sphygmomanometer, was introduced into to the United States at the turn of the twentieth century; however, another decade or two elapsed before the instrument was standardized and its use became a matter of routine.

[11]   W.M. Brown, "Reports of District Societies: Essex County," *TMSNJ* (1863): 54. Veratrum remained in use at the turn of the twentieth century and was mentioned by Osler for the treatment of pneumonia in his 1898 edition of his textbook; Osler, *Principles and Practice*, 135.

[12]   "On Veratrum Viride," *CP* 1, no. 1 (June 1879): 23; reprinted from the *Medical and Surgical Reporter*, no further citation. The editorial remarks on veratrum viride follow a brief letter from W. Sigsbee of Illinois to the *Medical and Surgical Reporter* and reprinted by Townsend; *CP* 1, no. 1 (June 1879): 22. The comments following Sigsbee's letter and quoted here appear to be written by EPT rather than the editor of the *Medical and Surgical Reporter*.

is now directed at the underlying lung disorder rather than the fast pulse. In severe cases with shock (in the modern use of the term), measures to enhance rather than diminish arterial tone are required. With successful treatment of the lung disease, the pulse returns to normal.

Townsend was particularly adamant that, in his fifteen years of practice, veratrum worked best in the early stages of pneumonia while the patient was still robust and "sthenic." Bloodletting left the patient, should he survive, anemic and weak, prolonging his convalescence and mandating the administration of tonics and stimulants. Was it not more reasonable, then, to relax the circulation pharmacologically and "save the circulating medium [blood] for further use."[13] Neither bloodletting nor veratrum were of any value "in the last stage when life is fast ebbing out . . . ."[14] In an editorial reprinted by Townsend from the *Medical and Surgical Reporter,* a veratrum enthusiast declared: " . . . so I would as soon think of leaving my house to see a patient without my hat, as without my little bottle of veratrum viride . . . ."[15]

In response to Gross' insistence on phlebotomy, Townsend trod carefully; he was in no position to challenge one of the leading physicians of Philadelphia, a surgeon and professor whose name was known throughout the country. The important thing—both he and Gross would agree—was not to trust pneumonia to "time and rosewater" (i.e., the healing powers of nature or *vis medicatrix naturae*). Much of the increased mortality of pneumonia and other inflammatory conditions, he concluded, was due to the "pusillanimity of medical men." Therapeutic skepticism was fashionable, but doing nothing beyond general supportive care was reckless and irresponsible. Townsend, as we know, was a veratrum man, but Gross and many of his readers favored phlebotomy or the administration of aconite (monkshood, another circulatory depressant). To such practitioners, Townsend said reassuringly: "every man works best with the implements he is most familiar with." The key thing was to do *something* to control

---

[13]   "On Veratrum Viride," 23.

[14]   EPT, "Double Pneumonia: Clinical Report of a Typical Case of Pneumonia," *CP* 2, no. 10 (March 1881): 326

[15]   "On Veratrum Viride," 23.

the circulation: " . . . when a physician is called to the bedside of a patient, suffering with an acute inflammatory affection, Professor Gross will agree with me it is the time to roll up his sleeves and fight for the life of the patient," whether it be with the lancet, veratrum viride, or aconite.[16]

It is difficult for us to imagine the terrors of diphtheria. During periodic epidemics, family physicians spent hours at the bedsides of dying children. Several siblings—all the children in a family—could die within days of one another, in some cases virtually strangled by obstruction of the upper airway by the classic diphtheric membrane. One of Townsend's favorite themes was the misdiagnosis and mistreatment of diphtheria. In 1876, he informed the Burlington County Medical Society that diphtheria was infrequent and overdiagnosed in his area; he himself had seen no recent cases. Many cases were in fact scarlet fever or other less ominous throat inflammations—and thus much more likely to resolve with any therapy (or no therapy). In many cases, "our homeopathic men report a great number of cases [of diphtheria], with miraculous cures."[17]

Townsend used the *Country Practitioner* to conduct what has come to be known as "collective research." Such research entailed the gathering of responses, usually by mail, to vexing medical questions by means of "circular letters"—a form of research by consensus designed to establish what we now call practice guidelines. Collective investigation did not challenge the status of the experienced practitioner as a legitimate source of medical authority.[18] In 1874, for example, members of the various county medical societies in New Jersey were asked by the state organization about their use of chloral hydrate and their personal experience with hypodermic medications.[19]

In the third issue of his journal, Townsend observed that a prominent Philadelphia "medical gentleman thinks a great

---

[16]   EPT, "Double Pneumonia," 325.

[17]   EPT, "Communication by Dr. Townsend," *TMSNJ* (1876): 182.

[18]   Harry M. Marks, *The Progress of Experiment: Science and Therapeutic Reform in the United States: 1900-1990* (Cambridge: Cambridge University Press, 1997), 43-44.

[19]   Frank Wilmarth, "Reports of District Societies: Essex County," *TMSNJ* (1874): 131-38.

benefit might accrue to the profession by a system of interviewing [by post]—in regard to medical questions." As a trial, he posed the following question: "Is diphtheria primarily, [sic] a local or constitutional affection?"[20] Unfortunately, the response was dismal. Townsend grumbled in the following issue: "Among the thousand and more recipients of our August number, no one seems to have any opinion in regard to the question asked . . . . or if so, they are too busy, too indifferent, or too lazy to answer."[21] Prompted by a case of diphtheria currently under his care "with very slight chance of recovery," Townsend tried another diphtheria questionnaire a few months later. No report of this survey was published in subsequent issues; most likely, there were few respondents.[22]

Even after Townsend left Beverly and moved on to Camden, New Jersey, in the late 1880s, he continued his crusade against poor medical practices in the diagnosis and management of diphtheria "by practitioners who never lost a case"—a cynical reference to incompetent sectarian practitioners and patent medicine hucksters who claimed extraordinary cures of misdiagnosed and overdiagnosed diphtheria. In Camden (1887), Townsend was involved in a tragic case of childhood diphtheria complicated by airway obstruction, hemorrhage, and cardiac decompensation.[23]

By the time diphtheria antitoxin, an early triumph of European microbiology laboratories and the germ theory of disease, was introduced in the 1890s, Townsend was practicing in Montana, still very much a frontier environment. For some years near the end of his life, he was an employee of the Indian Agency Service and must have seen many sick children and, almost certainly, there were cases of diphtheria on the reservations. It is unclear whether the new antitoxin serum was available on the western frontier; but having attended so many children dying of diphtheria in the course of his long career, there is little doubt that Townsend would have eagerly embraced the new antitoxin therapy.

---

20   [EPT], "Editorial," *CP* 1, no. 3 (August 1879): 107.
21   [EPT]; "Editorial," *CP* 1, no. 4 (September 1879): 143.
22   [EPT], "Please Answer the Following Questionnaire," *CP* 1, nos. 8,9 (January, February 1880): back covers.
23   John W. Snowden, "Reports of District Societies: Camden County," *TMSNJ* (1887): 313.

Obstetrics was an inevitable and often onerous part of country and village practice. Physicians strove to distinguish themselves from midwives, most of whom lacked any formal training, although some immigrant midwives arrived with excellent European training and others possessed sufficient intelligence and experience to save countless mothers and infants. Many graduates of American medical schools had little or no training in obstetrics; some had never delivered a baby prior to entering practice. As late as 1912, John Whitridge Williams of Johns Hopkins, a leading American obstetrician, bemoaned the deplorable state of American medical education in this field.[24] The years spent in military service during the Civil War by many young medical graduates of Townsend's generation did little to improve obstetric skills.

Obstetric practice, in all its aspects, made frequent appearances in the *Country Practitioner*. In general, medical journal articles on midwifery fell into two categories—the practical points of conducting a midwifery case and reports of complications. In the course of his career up until the mid-1890s, Townsend attended over twelve hundred obstetrical cases, most or all in the parturient's home.[25] In one case of prolonged labor described in detail in the *Country Practitioner*, Townsend and a colleague "exhausted about all the ether in the town." The physicians succeeded in delivering a dead fetus. The patient, thought to be suffering from "uremic poisoning" (kidney failure) and peritonitis, died six days later after numerous complications and almost continuous attendance by Townsend. The case, described in minute detail just a week or two after the event, clearly touched Townsend deeply and weighed heavily upon him.

The potential for censure from professional colleagues and friends of the patient, together with his own anxieties about the choices he made as the crisis unfolded, seem to the modern reader to be as profound a burden as the present threat of malpractice

---

[24]   John Whitridge Williams, "Medical Education and the Midwife Problem," *Journal of the American Medical Association* 58 (1912): 1-7.

[25]   EPT, "Back Alley Obstetrics," *Medical Sentinel* 2 (1894): 124-26. Townsend reported his experience with twelve hundred cases shortly after leaving New Jersey for Montana; it is clear from the context and the dates that most, if not all, of these cases were from his thirty years of practice in New Jersey.

litigation and the prospect of hospital departmental action and sanctions. Evidently in anguish over the loss of a laboring woman, Townsend wrote in the *Country Practitioner*:

> I quote this case only to show one of those horrible, harrowing positions into which the country physician is sometimes cast. Death at all times is terrible, but nowhere so much as in the lying-in chamber, and in country towns and villages, where every one is acquainted far and near, and the physician who attends must prepare to guard well his actions, and see that no room is left when all is over to reflect upon his treatment . . . . May each of my readers be spared a similar situation.[26]

Obstetrics was, for Townsend as for all practitioners of midwifery and obstetrics, hours of boredom punctuated by moments of terror. The theme of obstetrics as a professional minefield was again taken up in the last issue of the *Country Practitioner*, published in September, 1881. Townsend urged his readers to be *au courant* and alert to potential complications. A list of "Obstetric Aphorisms" borrowed from the *Michigan Medical News* included the warning: "Cleanliness is especially next to godliness in the case of the accoucheur. Its absence renders one liable to professional homicide."[27]

On a more quotidian level, readers of the *Country Practitioner* were brought up to date by two articles on a vexing obstetrical issue of the day: the pros and cons of bandaging (binding) the abdomen after labor and delivery.[28] One contributor cited the good results of a celebrated Parisian midwife (along with African and Indian women) who eschewed bandaging.[29] The proper use of obstetrical forceps, a symbol of the "male midwife" was covered in an article reprinted from *American Journal of Medicine*.[30]

---

[26] [EPT], "Leaves from the Diary of a Country Doctor," *CP* 2, no. 10 (March 1881): 330.

[27] H. Webster Jones, "Obstetric Aphorisms," *CP* 3, no. 3 (September 1881): 115.

[28] Alexander Elwell, "Should We Bandage after Labor and Why?" *CP* 1, no. 12 (May 1880): 417-19.

[29] Hiram Corson, "Post-partum Binders," *CP* 2, no. 5 (October 1880): 149-52.

[30] A.J. Howe, "When Obstetrical Forceps Are to Be Used," *CP* 2, no. 12 (May 1881): 416-77; reprinted from the *American Medical Journal*, St. Louis, no further

Guidelines on the use of forceps were also provided in succinct form in an article reprinted from the *Obstetrical Journal.*[31]

In addition to the medical challenges of pregnancy, the country practitioner was forced to cope with interfering neighbors who cluttered up the lying-in chamber and sick-rooms in general, offering ill-informed advice and undermining the expertise and authority of the physician. In his younger days, when he was afraid of offending prospective patients and had not yet acquired backbone, Townsend claimed to have had "frequent cases of puerperal fever brought on by half a dozen women gossiping in the lying-in chamber. That time is past, and the visitor that enters such a chamber under my control at the present time never cares to repeat the offense."[32]

In an article published in 1894, months after he left New Jersey for Montana, Townsend mentioned his experience in twelve hundred obstetrical cases, probably an estimate of the total deliveries he had attended in the course of his thirty-year career in New Jersey, both in Beverly and later on in the larger city of Camden. His article, which appeared in the *Medical Sentinel*, a northwestern medical journal published from 1893 in Portland, Oregon, was titled "Back Alley Obstetrics." By "back alley," Townsend meant poor homes with little or no hygiene, rather than the more ominous modern reference to illegal abortion.

Through much of the nineteenth century, the issue of "meddlesome midwifery," often equated with "male midwifery" or the replacement of traditional female midwives by physicians in the birthing room, was a subject of much debate in American obstetrics. Even before the germ theory of disease was widely accepted, physicians came to realize that they themselves might transfer infectious matter to parturient women in the course of

---

citation.

[31] Barnes, "General Conclusions in Regard to the Use of Forceps," *CP* 1, no. 7 (December 1879), 248; reprinted from *Obstetrical Journal*, no further citation.

[32] EPT, "Notes and Comments: Sick Room Visitations," *CP* 2, no. 6 (November 1880): 192. It is unlikely that clusters of visitors who did not actually examine the patient would transmit puerperal fever; the hands of the midwife and physician(s), who would have conducted internal examination, were probably at fault.

examination and instrumentation.[33] Midwives, whether skilled or unskilled, washed or unwashed, did not use forceps and in many cases performed very limited internal examinations. Oliver Wendell Holmes of Boston met with violent opposition from colleagues in 1843 when he charged them with carrying infectious material from autopsies on their hands and clothing, subsequently transmitting puerperal sepsis ("childbed fever") to laboring women, often with a fatal outcome. Townsend was most likely aware of Holmes' essay and the work of Ignaz Semmelweiss (published 1861), a Hungarian physician working in Vienna, who demonstrated statistically that women in a large public lying-in hospital were far less likely to die of puerperal sepsis if attended by midwives rather than by physicians. Physicians in the Vienna hospital, in their quest to understand the cause of the appalling maternal mortality, routinely performed autopsies on women who died of puerperal sepsis. Without changing clothing or washing their hands, they returned to the crowded wards, carrying the fatal bacteria with them from woman to woman. When Semmelweiss instituted strict handwashing in an antiseptic solution, the mortality rate fell precipitously in the lying-in wards of the Vienna hospital. Holmes' essay and Semmelweiss' brilliant demonstration preceded the germ theory, which gained traction in the 1870s. Strict handwashing and other aseptic and antiseptic precautions by midwives and physicians would not become standard for several decades.

In reviewing his own experience with home rather than hospital delivery, Townsend, like Semmelweiss and Holmes, reached a disturbing and counterintuitive conclusion. In the squalid dwellings of "back alleys" wrote Townsend, the physician finds his patient "in a filthy bed, dressed in filthy clothing, and [is] lucky if it [i.e., the bed] does not contain more living things than [i.e., in addition to] the patient." Nevertheless, Townsend observed that most such women did well and their infants survived.

---

[33] Holmes' paper, "On the Contagiousness of Puerperal Fever," was read at the Boston Society for Medical Improvement in 1843 and subsequently published in the *New England Quarterly Journal for Medicine and Surgery* 1 (1843). See Logan Clendening, *Source Book of Medical History* (New York: Henry Schuman, 1942; reprinted New York: Dover, 1960), 603-6. The full text of Holmes' paper is online at http://www.bartleby.com/38/5/1.html (accessed July 2, 2010).

How could this be explained? While many poor women were attended by female midwives, middle class and wealthy women were increasingly turning to formally trained physicians, who were, of course, mostly male. In accordance with their training, physicians conducted frequent examinations and inserted forceps into the uterine cavity to hasten a difficult delivery. The use of "high forceps" has disappeared from modern obstetrical practice, but was common prior to the routinization of Caesarian delivery. Such "meddlesome midwifery is mischievous," wrote Townsend, and promoted septicemia (childbed fever).[34] The implied criticism of some of his colleagues was self-evident and none too subtle. It was his belief that normally progressing labor required little or no intervention. Trusting to nature, with active intervention only when absolutely necessary, seemed the safest course in Townsend's view:

> The duty of the obstetrician, who is in general practice (three times out of four an emergency man), is to always be personally clean, go to his patient, diagnose the case, and then stand by to assist nature if she needs it, but otherwise to interfere as little as possible.[35]

Gynecology was, of course, also the province of the country practitioner. On the subject of diagnosing ovarian cysts in those years before diagnostic imaging, one of Townsend's colleagues from Burlington County mused: "The diagnostician attempting to attack scylla too often meets shipwreck on charybdis . . . ."[36]

A far more controversial issue was Battey's operation. "Ovariotomy," or the removal of both healthy ovaries (i.e., surgical castration, more correctly oophorectomy) was introduced in America in 1872 by Georgia surgeon Robert Battey. The operation was widely adopted for a range of functional, physical, and "nervous"

---

[34] EPT, "Back Alley Obstetrics," 124, 126.

[35] Ibid., 125.

[36] R.H. Page, "Report of Case from *Transactions of the Burlington County Medical Society*," *CP* 2, no. 1 (June 1880): 4. Scylla and Charybdis (uncapitalized in *CP*) were sea monsters guarding opposite shores of the narrow straits of Messina in Greek myth; to be between Scylla and Charybdis meant that danger was unavoidable.

symptoms, the latter including hysteria and nymphomania. The theory behind such surgery rested on seemingly scientific theories of reflex irritation, which held that all the organs of the body were connected by neural pathways through the spinal cord, which functioned as a sort of switching stations.[37] The female organs were obvious targets of medical concern within the paradigms of reflex irritation. It seemed logical that many vague disorders affecting women should respond to such interventions as non-surgical repositioning of the "tilted" uterus by the insertion of vaginal pessaries. Small-town general practitioners, as well as urban specialists, embraced Battey's operation for several decades before it fell out of favor. Surgical mortality varied, but was far from trivial. Townsend selected an article from the *North Carolina Medical Journal* for his readers. The author "and other distinguished authorities" dismissed the notion that castration in young women "completely obliterates all desire for sexual congress" and robs the young woman of her charms. Furthermore, the strictest adherence to the antiseptic principles and practices of Joseph Lister, as applied scrupulously by the author of the paper, much reduced the risk of postoperative septicemia and death.[38]

Aside from obstetrics and gynecology, other issues of the day that captured Townsend's attention included the merits of bromide of ethyl as an anesthetic (claimed by some to be superior to ether and chloroform) and the perennial indifference to smallpox vaccination among the population.[39] From the *Proceedings of the Medical Society of Kings* came a third-hand article originally published by the State Board of Health of Michigan titled "Treatment of the Drowned."[40] Following a common practice among American medical journals of the day, Townsend occasionally reprinted

---

[37] Edward Shorter, *From Paralysis to Fatigue* (New York: Free Press, 1992), 40, 73-79.

[38] T.B. Wilkerson, "Removal of Both Ovaria, or 'Battey's Operation' for the Cure of Insanity," *CP* 3, no. 2 (August 1881): 56-61.

[39] [EPT], "Notes and Comments: Anaesthetics," *CP* 1, no. 12 (May 1880): 425-6; Hiram Corson, "On Small-Pox," *CP* 3, no. 3 (September 1881): 81-86.

[40] "Treatment of the Drowned," *CP* 1, no. 6 (November 1879): 192-95; reprinted from *Proceedings of the Medical Society, County of Kings*, which reprinted the article from the State Board of Health of Michigan, no further citation.

a lecture from a respected medical school professor. "On the Therapeutics of Rheumatism" by Roberts Bartholow, professor of therapeutics and materia medica (study of medications and their administration, since replaced by the discipline of pharmacology) at Jefferson Medical College in Philadelphia, was one such essay.[41]

The *Country Practitioner* served as something of a soapbox for Townsend. Like many editors, he did not hesitate to push his agenda, not only in medical matters such as the use of veratrum and the proper diagnosis of diphtheria, but in all aspects of medical practice. Medicine was hailed as a noble calling, but it was also the major source of income for the physician and his family. In the nineteenth century, medical practice paid poorly and often erratically for all but the most elite urban consultants. Irregular sectarian practitioners were not only an affront to the self-image of a dignified medical brotherhood, but also a nagging source of competition for patient patronage. Practicing among friends and neighbors had its rewards, although the business aspects presented an added source of friction and discontent. The following chapter examines these issues as they were presented in the pages of the *Country Practitioner*.

---

[41] Roberts Bartholow, "On the Therapeutics of Acute Rheumatism," *CP* 1, no. 10 (March 1880): 325-31; reprinted from *Medical News and Abstract*, no further citation.

CHAPTER 7

THE VIEW FROM BEVERLY:

THE BUSINESS AND ETHICS OF MEDICINE

From the first issue, the *Country Practitioner* tried to define the proper code of conduct for physicians and provided a forum for addressing some of the troubling aspects of the business of medicine. The status of organized medicine, particularly with respect to state licensing, was a topic upon which New Jersey physicians expended much ink during the course of the nineteenth century. Townsend's *Country Practitioner* predictably took the American Medical Association line, denigrating the lay practitioners and healing cultists who practiced medicine, often quite successfully in terms of income, without a proper medical school degree. Jacksonian sensibilities and the cult of the common man extended only so far; the watchword of the regular medical profession was licensing, or at least credentialing. In an editorial in March, 1881, Townsend reprinted an amendment to an act of the New Jersey legislature titled "An Act to Regulate the Practice of Medicine and Surgery." Practicing without proper registration would be punishable by a fine of twenty-five dollars and imprisonment for up to six months for each professional encounter or prescription. However, to Townsend's chagrin, the bill also stated that "any person who shall have had twenty years experience in the practice of medicine or surgery in one locality shall be exempt from the provisions of this act." Thus, "old quacks" seem to have been given a pass. Townsend fumed: "We reprint the above amendment to the Medical Registration Act simply to show how the Senate and House of Representatives of a State may be suborned to the interests of the lowest and most despicable of imposters."[1] Similar editorials appeared over the course of the nineteenth century in local, state, and regional medical journals.

Indeed, the major practice issue through much of the nineteenth century was the quest for licensing laws and some measure of control over the irregular practitioners who competed for patients in what has come to be called the medical marketplace. Townsend jumped right into the fray. In an editorial entitled "Wanted—Backbone," Townsend made his case for licensing laws and used his old nemesis, James Still, as an example, driving his point home with a New Jersey metaphor: "One hoary-headed old negro in Burlington County—who knows no more about medicine than a Barnegat clam—defies the law."[2] In 1881, Townsend characterized Still, whom he referred to as "the Ethiopian salve doctor," as "[a]n Artful Dodger . . . who has amassed a fortune from the gullible people of West Jersey and adjacent parts." Townsend accused Still of "persistent stupidity," and held his herbal practice up as an example of the dangers of continued dithering by state legislators on the issue of licensing legislation.[3] Although his salves and herbs and lack of any formal training may have placed him outside the medical brotherhood, Still was anything but "stupid," as his autobiography amply demonstrates.[4]

Until the end of the nineteenth century, regular physicians conveniently lumped all sectarians (including homeopaths and eclectics, many of whom had attended legitimate sectarian schools with courses of study comparable to regular medical colleges) under the category of "quacks." A contributor to *The Country Practitioner* from New Jersey's rural Gloucester County railed

---

[1] [EPT], "Editorial," *CP* 2, no. 10 (March 1881): 354.

[2] [EPT], "Wanted—Backbone," *CP* 2, no. 5 (October 1880): 158. Barnegat Bay is on the Atlantic coast of New Jersey and was once the site of an active clamming industry.

[3] Ellis P. Townsend, "An Artful Dodger," *CP* 2, no. 9 (February 1881): 294-95.

[4] James Still: *Early Recollections and Life of James Still* (Philadelphia: J.B. Lippincott, 1877).

against "bogus colleges and their clinical backers." His call to arms took something of a vigilante tone:

> Turn the profession loose upon these vampires, untie their hands that they may also hurl back missiles and mud if necessary and these miscreants who are preying upon the credulity of the country, will in turn be driven to cover . . . . Think it over boys and let's charge the whole line, I believe we can knock them into smithereens.[5]

By the turn of the century, New Jersey had been home to at least three such fraudulent institutions: Livingston University in Haddonfield, Hygeio-Therapeutic College in Bergen Heights or Florence (see note), and the College of Fine Forces in East Orange, all non-operational as of 1896.[6] Livingston University, a bogus diploma mill operating in the 1860s from a farm in Haddonfield in Camden County, was better known as the University of Medicine and Surgery of Haddonfield. The Haddonfield operation was but one of dozens of fraudulent diploma mills operated by the notorious John Buchanan, a quondam professor of eclectic medicine. At the time of his arrest in Philadelphia, Buchanan admitted to issuing tens of thousands of fake diplomas through various fraudulent medical and dental schools.[7] Townsend took

[5]   J. Down Heritage, "The Medical Profession," *CP* 2, no. 2 (July 1880): 42.

[6]   R.L. Polk, ed., *Medical and Surgical Register of the United States*, 4th ed. rev. (Detroit, Chicago: R.L. Polk & Co., 1896), 118. The Polk register's stated location of the Hygieo-Therapeutic College in Bergen Heights is confusing. The Hygieo-Therapeutic College was the name of Russell T. Trall's hydropathic treatment and training institute in Florence Heights (Burlington County), operating from 1869 to 1875. See Sandra Moss, "Fountains of Youth: New Jersey Water-Cures," *Garden State Legacy* 1(2) (2008), online at GardenStateLegacy.com (access limited to subscribers). The Medical and Surgical College of the State of New Jersey, Jersey City, appeared to be an eclectic medical school, with most of its faculty in New York. It was incorporated in 1880, and its charter repealed in 1891 by the New Jersey Board of Medical Examiners; "Repeal of Charter of the Medical and Surgical College of New Jersey—New Jersey State Board of Medical Examiners," *Boston Medical and Surgical Journal* 124 (1891): 299. No graduates were listed in the medical directories of the day.

[7]   "Buchanan Gives Up the Fight: Charters of Two of the Bogus Medical Colleges Annulled," *New York Times*, October 1, 1880; David L. Cowen, *Medicine and Health in New Jersey: A History* (Princeton: D. Van Nostrand, 1964), 76-7; William J. Snape,

up the topic of diploma mills in an editorial entitled "Bogus Diplomas," in which he referred to the "swindlers" recently hunted down in Philadelphia, a probable reference to Buchanan.[8] The Burlington County Medical Society was aware of "seven cases of Buchanan Diplomas" registered with the county clerk (as was required of all medical diplomas whether "regular" or sectarian) at Mount Holly.[9]

Townsend and A.W. Taylor, his fellow regular physician in Beverly, had some local competition from the irregulars. H.J. Roberts, M.D., who practiced as a "homoeopathist" and advertised himself as "successor to Dr. C.R. Cloud," had a practice in Beverly in the 1870s.[10] As a homeopathic practitioner, Roberts would not have been listed in the *Medical Register* and would not have been admitted into the Burlington County Medical Society. Townsend, judging from comments in *The Country Practitioner*, had little respect for homeopaths and would not have consulted with Robert; at that time, such consultation with "irregulars" was proscribed by the Code of Ethics of the American Medical Association. Additional competition for Townsend and Taylor came from the patent medicine hucksters. The *Beverly Weekly Visitor* not only listed the addresses and hours of the physicians, a dentist, and a druggist in its "Business Card" section, but also promoted such products as "Barbeur's Russian Remedy," a cure for cancer, erysipelas (bacterial skin infection), and scrofula (a form of tuberculosis of the lymph nodes).[11]

"The Rise and Fall of John Buchanan 'M.D.': Founder of Livingstone University, Haddonfield, N.J.," *Bulletin of the Camden County Historical Society* 24 (1970): 17-19.

[8] [EPT], "Bogus Diplomas," *CP* 2, no. 1 (June 1880) 32-33.

[9] *Burlington County Medical Society Minute Book: 1869-1893* (entry October 13, 1880).

[10] "Business Cards," *Beverly Weekly Visitor*, June 15, 1878. Roberts, the homeopathic physician, was included in the "Business Cards" listing in the *Beverly Weekly Visitor*. Listing of regular physicians in Beverly confirmed through review of pertinent issues of Alfred E.M. Purdy (ed.) succeeded by Wm. H. White (ed.), *The Medical Registry of New York, New Jersey, and Connecticut* (New York, G.P. Putnam's Sons), issued annually. Date of Taylor's graduation from medical school, "List of Physicians," *CP*, 2, no. 3 (August, 1880): 79-80.

[11] "Local Matter," *Beverly Weekly Visitor*, November 10, 1877. American Medical Association, *Code of Medical Ethics of the American Medical Association*, (Chicago:

The waiving or reduction of fees for other physicians, and often their families, was routine and unquestioned until recently. Men of God presented a more difficult challenge. In colonial America, clergymen, as the most educated men in the community, often provided medical advice; some had studied medicine in Europe before coming to America. Townsend added his voice to that of other journal editors who took on, none too delicately, the delicate issue of professional courtesy to clergymen. Townsend intoned, "Indeed, it is a reproach to our civilization to have a privileged class whose only claim to consideration in financial matters is that they are ministers of the gospel." Physicians, after all, supported churches and ministers with tithes and contributions and, as a profession, provided free care for charitable cases. Moreover, it was irritating to regular physicians that "clergymen, as a class, give to quackery in medicine more countenance and support, than any other class of citizens of equal intelligence, while they expect to be attended free by the regular profession."[12]

The *Country Practitioner* reprinted an editorial from the *Chicago Medical Gazette* with the ominous title, "The Clergy Must Pay." The Chicago editor thundered: "Thousands of ministers think they have a right divine to live more cheaply than other people, and to be sick without cost to themselves." Ministers, who were, after all, paid "living salaries . . . . ought to live on them." And, to add insult to injury, the quacks so warmly embraced by ministers expected to be paid and never extended professional courtesy.[13] Clearly, these borrowed articles struck a chord with Townsend, who reprinted them without caveat or apology.

Worse yet, busybody clergymen were often a positive menace in the sick room. A second item from the *Chicago Gazette*

American Medical Association Press, 1847), 98. Full text of the 1847 *Code of Medical Ethics of the American Medical Association* is reproduced online at http://www.ama-assn.org/ama1/pub/upload/mm/369/1847code.pdf (accessed December 2, 2010). The section on consultation appears in chapter 2, article 4, paragraph 1: "But no one can be considered as a regular practitioner, or a fit associate in consultation whose practice is based on an exclusive dogma, to the rejection of the accumulated experience of the profession . . . ."

[12]　[EPT], "Gratuitous Services to Clergymen," *CP* 1, no. 8 (January 1880): 264.

[13]　"The Clergy Must Pay," *CP* 1, no. 12 (May 1880): 433; reprinted from *Chicago Medical Gazette*, no further citation.

attributed sickroom clashes between clergy and physicians to the "bearishness of the physician, the stupidity of the clergyman, or both. By the very necessities of his profession the physician must have authority in the sick room."[14] Included in the same class as busybody clergymen were busybody know-it-all neighbors in the sick room or lying-in room. Townsend insisted, "Every physician who values the lives of his patients, or his own reputation, should constitute himself the sergeant-at-arms of the sick room, issue his positive orders and see that they are carried out."[15]

How these editorials impacted Townsend's relation with the local clergy is not clear. Some years before starting his medical journal, Townsend, in his pamphlet, *Suburban Homes*, took note of the "fine churches" in Beverly.[16] Clergymen would not have subscribed to the *Country Practitioner*, but one of Townsend's Burlington County medical colleagues might have shown one or two of the editorials to his own clergyman—in that case, the word would have spread quickly through the clerical grapevine. If Townsend had a falling-out with the local pastors on the issue, there is no record of the fact. His medical colleagues, whatever their public posture, probably uttered a silent "amen." Medical practice did not pay well and collections were often difficult; a lifetime of free care for clergymen and possibly their families could not but create resentment. Townsend apparently did not take his incendiary views on professional courtesy to clergymen with him to Montana when he left New Jersey in 1893. He died in the good graces of the Presbyterian Church in Billings, where the Reverend B.Z. McCullough "delivered a touching tribute."[17]

The business of medicine was a constant concern in an era when country physicians struggled to squeeze a living out of medical practice. Like most medical journal editors, Townsend editorialized on practice issues. For the majority of his subscribers,

---

[14]   "Clergymen in the Sick Room," *CP* 2, no. 1 (June 1881): 29; reprinted from *Chicago Medical Gazette*, no further citation.

[15]   EPT, "Sick Room Visitations," *CP* 2, no. 6 (November 1880): 192.

[16]   EPT, *Suburban Homes* (ca. 1874), 2.

[17]   *Forsyth Times*, August 8, 1907 (untitled obituary and funeral notice); photocopy courtesy Montana State Historical Society.

medical practice was only moderately remunerative, often wearying, and occasionally confrontational.

In Townsend's view, country doctors did little to help themselves in the matter of income. Soft of heart and restrained by the "sympathy they acquire at the bedside of the suffering," physicians were, in general, "miserable book keepers and cowardly collectors." Office patients should be made to pay on the spot! There was, moreover, no excuse for lack of payment of obstetric fees. After all, argued Townsend, the new father "has known for nine months that the services would be required and the customary fee should be ready" to hand the doctor before he leaves the house where he has provided obstetric services.[18] "If the practitioner does not place any value on his own services no one will do it for him," intoned Townsend. He suggested that doctors might learn something from "the legal fraternity" in setting prices and making collections.[19]

Townsend seemed to possess a wry sense of humor. In advising young men about to enter into country practice (buy a horse, marry well to a wealthy local woman with plenty of relatives prepared to sing your praises, and cultivate the ministers), he ended this tongue-in-cheek editorial with wise advice about the older practitioners in the community. The "old fogies," with their well-established practices, may not be up on the latest medical theories and practices, but they knew a thing or two that might help the new young medical man in town. And they knew how to retain the loyalty of their patients.[20]

The iconic image of the old country doctor—riding alone for miles through fence-high snowdrifts and raging storms—was no myth. Two tales of perilous rides were recalled in "Leaves from the Diary of a Country Doctor" in the final number of the second volume. In one case "T" (possibly Townsend) rode through heavy snowdrifts to an exsanguinating woman with a stillborn infant—truly an emergency. In the second case he and a servant risked a carriage ride through a terrifying thunderstorm to respond to an urgent call and a demand that he not delay until

---

18   [EPT], "Editorial," *CP* 2, no. 11 (April 1881): 387.
19   [EPT], "Editorial," *CP* 1, no. 4 (September 1879): 141.
20   [EPT], "Practice Hunters," *CP* 2, no. 11 (April 1881): 366-67.

after the storm had passed. Upon arrival, he "expected to find a desperate case," only to learn that the mother insisted he check her "ruddy, healthy-looking urchin of twelve years," for worms! His temper was "not altogether serene."[21]

Isolation, a particular concern for the country practitioner, was countered by the natural and universal tendency to form professional societies. The Medical Society of New Jersey, founded in 1766, announced that among its goals was "cultivating the utmost harmony and friendship with their Brethren. . . ."[22] Medical societies enhanced the meager political influence of the regular profession as well as providing a forum for discussion of cases and what has come to be called continuing medical education. The state society met but a year, and few rural physicians had the time, funds, or inclination to attend regularly. The Burlington County Medical Society met quarterly. Despite the difficulties of crossing the large rural county, some dozen members, including Townsend, clearly valued the professional camaraderie. Unlike Townsend, many physicians made little or no effort to keep up with medical progress, either through reading journals or engaging in professional discourse with colleagues. In the absence of state licensing legislation, nothing could be done to discipline such physicians. However, the *Country Practitioner* did not hesitate to chastise men whose education had halted decades early with the completion of medical school or apprenticeship.

---

[21]   T, "Leaves from the Diary of a Country Doctor," *CP* 2, no. 12 (May 1881): 397. From context, this was probably authored by Townsend, although most unsigned work in *CP* does not bear his initial(s).

[22]   Stephen Wickes, *The Rise, Minutes, and Proceedings of the New Jersey Medical Society, Established July 23d, 1766* (Newark: Jennings & Hardham, 1875), 4.

CHAPTER 8

THE PROFESSIONAL BROTHERHOOD

Townsend was an organization man when it came to the professional brotherhood of regular physicians. He was a member of his county and state medical societies, as well as a member of the American Medical Association. Although the *Transactions of the Medical Society of New Jersey* was published annually, Townsend commented on important issues related to New Jersey's county and state medical societies in the pages of the *Country Practitioner*. This was not inconsistent with his goal of a national readership. Physicians across the country concerned themselves with issues such as licensing and quackery.

Townsend was not intimidated by the windy rhetoric and scientific proceedings of state and national medical associations. In fact, he did not hesitate to express his rather low opinion of their meetings and publications. The 1880 meeting of the Medical Society of New Jersey was held in Princeton. In Townsend's view, the "regular essays were hurriedly read to almost empty seats, a number of volunteer papers were crowded out, and no time was had for questions or discussions on the papers presented."[1] In 1881, the meeting was held in Long Branch on New Jersey's Atlantic shore, where the hotel was "a disgrace to the proprietors and to Long Branch, the tables were badly served, the material

---

[1] Ellis P. Townsend, "New Jersey State Medical Society," *CP* 2, no. 1 (June 1880): 11.

deficient in quantity and quality and the prices outrageous." Attendees claimed it was "the poorest meeting held by the Society for thirty years." Physicians, observed Townsend, "care very little what they pay if properly served."[2]

In 1881, he held forth on the American Medical Association, "this great unwieldy body," and the "ponderous edition of its transactions." Its scientific session "accomplished nothing of value," and any physician "who will scrutinize the published transactions of the American Medical or of the State Medical societies will be convinced that the majority of the papers presented are of such a character that they would be consigned to the waste basket of a medical publisher."[3]

Most New Jersey physicians who "kept up" did so through local, county, and statewide societies. One or two delegates were appointed by the Medical Society of New Jersey to report on out-of-state meetings; these reports appeared in the annual *Transactions of the Medical Society of New Jersey*. Such emissaries added little to the fund of medical knowledge in the state. Townsend himself had submitted such a report to the Burlington County Medical Society in 1866 following a meeting of the state society in New Brunswick; he noted only that "the meeting was very interesting—that their was much [?unclear handwritng] to instruct, and that the members generally seemed much gratified."[4] A colleague's report to the Medical Society of New Jersey regarding an 1879 meeting of the Pennsylvania State Medical Society in 1879 called forth similar bromides: "The meeting was very harmonious . . . . There were fifteen essays and papers read . . . . The papers and essays were of unusual interest, and I regret in this brief report I cannot refer separately to them."[5]

Townsend challenged the state and national medical organizations to raise their standards of medical education and

---

2   [EPT], "Society Transactions: State Medical Society of New Jersey," *CP* 3, no. 1 (July 1881): 8.

3   [EPT], "Society Transactions: American Medical Association." *CP* 3, no. 1 (July 1881): 3.

4   *Secretary's Book: Burlington County Medical Society* (entry April 10, 1866).

5   H. Genet Taylor, "Report of the Delegate to the Pennsylvania State Medical Society," *TMSNJ* (1879): 34.

make meetings worth the time, travel, and expense involved. As delegate from New Jersey to the Pennsylvania society meeting in 1880, however, Townsend resorted to the usual boilerplate about interesting and "valuable" papers, cordial welcomes, and society business. More usefully, he devoted the balance of his brief report to registering his frustration with rambling meetings, and lauded efforts by the Pennsylvania society to limit addresses to twenty minutes (thirty for the president) and discussion to thirty minutes. He chastised his New Jersey colleagues for over-lengthy presentations that could benefit from "curtailment and condensation," pointing out that papers and reports "are not valued by their length . . . ."[6]

Townsend lamented the failure of many physicians to keep abreast of medical progress and improve their medical knowledge and skills. Doubtless, he agreed with J.W., a contributor to the *Country Practitioner*. In a feisty and somewhat damning article, Hickman was critical of colleagues who made no effort to keep current. Hickman, of course, was preaching to the choir, and he stood little risk of antagonizing the non-reading targets of his article. Experience and a dimly remembered medical education, wrote Hickman, were not enough to mark the good physician, but instead led to "undue self-confidence" when unaccompanied by "earnest diligence in study and research." Rather, colleagues should look to his journals and books to see if he keeps up; look to his careful records of cases and his "earnest diligence." It was "a deplorable fact that a majority of medical men are idlers in the way of improving themselves." More often than not, such men used just a few drugs, and then poorly. "Their knowledge of medicine is absolute empiricism, and their experience but a mockery and even a shame." The clinical thermometer was rejected by some of the older practitioners, "confident that years of practice have enabled them to become sufficiently well trained in eye and touch to dispense with more accurate aid in this direction." The same held true for urinalysis. "We truthfully sum up the matter by repeating that thickly-strewn, in city and country alike, are the practitioners

---

6   EPT, "Report of Delegate to State Medical Society of Pennsylvania," *TMSNJ* (1880): 32-33.

who know shamefully little of what has been done in the way of advancing medical knowledge since the day of their graduation. Their diploma protects them from the law, and thus they go on, a drag and tether to the profession." And the price they exact, cautioned Hickman, is the "sacrifice of human life."[7]

A most valuable and original contribution to *The Country Practitioner* was a case flow chart designed by J. Down Heritage, a physician from Glassboro in adjacent rural Gloucester County. Included on the chart were sections for the patient's history and physical examination, progress and nursing notes, and prescriptions and treatment plans. Heritage stressed that universal use of such a form would turn the state medical society into a "clinic" in which success and failure in battling disease could be reliably assessed. He concluded:

> I am, therefore, fully persuaded from my own experience that a fair trial of the blank . . . will be a source of gratification to the physician, an incentive to accurate effort, an incitement to keep abreast [sic] the advancement of our science, will be an admirable educator, and once adopted will be persevered in, at least in severe cases and epidemics.[8]

Townsend, in an accompanying editorial, lauded the form and suggested "dotting out" (graphing) the daily readings of temperature, pulse, and urinary output. Despite the extra work involved, " . . . only those [practitioners] who keep themselves in the advance guard of true medical progress can expect success." Townsend, who seems to have lost some of his confidence in his fellow country practitioners, expected that "the majority of the older members of the profession will undoubtedly pooh-pooh" Heritage's form and "pronounce it supremely ridiculous.[9]

---

7   J.W. Hickman, "The Value of Experience in the Practice of Medicine," *CP*, 1, no 8 (January 1880): 254, 255.

8   J. Down Heritage, "Clinical Reports in Private Practice," *CP* 1, no. 11 (April 1880): 370. The Gloucester County Medical Society, organized 1881, had but six members in 1881: "Members of District Medical Societies," *TMSNJ* (1881): 13.

9   [EPT], "Editorial," *CP* 1, no. 11 (April 1880): 399.

Many practitioners of the day kept, at best, brief notes indicating little more than the diagnosis and prescribed treatment. Sketchy clinical notes were often entered into ledger books, along with dates of attendance and details of fee collection. Some intellectually curious physicians constructed detailed longitudinal records of obstetrical cases or other medical encounters of personal interest. For example, in Bordentown (Burlington County), Dr. Irene Dupont Young kept a detailed tabulation of obstetrical cases from 1849 to 1880.[10] Hospitals were beginning to institute standard charting procedures, but few general physicians would have considered such a form practical in their domestic and office practices.[11] Practitioners who performed insurance examinations for one or more companies would have been familiar with printed forms by the 1870s; the medical director of each company prepared detailed forms to shape the examination and standardize reporting.[12] However, such forms did not routinely carry over into office practice. While it is likely that few if any readers adopted Heritage's form, both Heritage and Townsend were thinking well ahead of their contemporaries in private practice.

Generalists such as Townsend and, indeed, most country and small town practitioners, felt themselves increasingly under siege. Not only was it well nigh impossible to keep up with advances in every field of medicine, but patients were coming

---

[10]   Irene Dupont Young, *Obstetric Register,"* (1849-1880), University of Medicine and Dentistry of New Jersey Special Collections, Newark, New Jersey. While he was apparently named for someone in the DuPont family of Delaware, in which the name Irénée appears in several generations, there is no evidence that Young was connected to that family. The spelling "Irene" was used in the county medical society membership lists published in the *TMSNJ*.

[11]   The use of forms in hospitals was an early twentieth-century phenomenon. See Joel D. Howell, *Technology in the Hospital: Transforming Patient Care in the Early Twentieth Century* (Baltimore: Johns Hopkins University Press, 1995), 45-8. For examples of the scope of hospital records in urban northern hospitals, see John Harley Warner, *The Therapeutic Perspective: Medical Practice, Knowledge, and Identity in America, 1820-1885* (Princeton: Princeton University Press: 1997), 84-85, 102-3.

[12]   For an overview of the state of the art of insurance examination in the late nineteenth century, see John M. Keating, *How to Examine for Life Insurance* (Philadelphia: WB Saunders, 1891). Keating includes sample forms from several dozen large life insurance companies. Keating was president of the Association of Life Insurance Medical Directors.

to expect (or demand) referrals to urban specialists. While some saw specialization as an opportunity, others saw it as a threat to reputation and income. Townsend and his contributors grappled with this thorny issue in the pages of the *Country Practitioner*.

CHAPTER 9

THE THREAT OF SPECIALIZATION AND OTHER
TOPICS OF THE DAY

One of the problems facing country doctors, whose stock in trade was their facility as generalists, was the rise of specialties in nearby cities. In an informal way, general physicians had long recognized that some of their colleagues, while continuing to attend to the full range of patients, were naturally more gifted and dexterous in surgical practice, while others possessed sharper diagnostic skills and still others were better prepared to cope with obstetrical emergencies. More than a few would-be specialists were eager to abandon such staples of general practice as obstetrics, which ate up their time and disrupted the smooth turnover of patients during house-call rounds and office hours. Some doctors gravitated naturally to dexterity-intense fields such as surgery, while others liked fiddling with the new diagnostic devices that proliferated after mid-century in fields such as ophthalmology, otolaryngology, and urology.

Medical knowledge, once quite static, expanded rapidly after the Civil War. Clearly, the individual physician could no longer master the bodies of knowledge and sets of skills that made up the new universe of medical theory and practice. Although country doctors of necessity continued as generalists, urban physicians, particularly the elite, gravitated toward specialization. In their world of medical colleges, high-profile private clientele, and journal publications, specialization brought prestige and, for many, relative wealth.

The American Medical Association had initially aligned itself with the general practitioners. Beginning in the 1860s, however, the national organization increasingly recognized specialties by creating special "sections." For example, the Section on Obstetrics and Gynecology appeared in 1860, and the Section on Ophthalmology, Otology, and Laryngology in the 1870s. Academies such as the New York Academy of Medicine also formed specialty sections. Urban, regional, and national specialty societies sprang up; national meetings and subspecialty journals soon followed. In the 1860s, the American Otological Society and the American Ophthalmology Society were organized. In the 1870s, the American Laryngological Association and the American Gynecological Society appeared. The 1880s saw the founding of the American Association of Genito-Urinary Surgeons, the American Orthopedic Association, and the American Association of Obstetricians and Gynecologists.[1] Medical school curricula, not surprisingly, became increasingly fragmented.[2] Professors, once drawn from the ranks of general practitioners with an interest in a particular area (such as surgery or anatomy), identified themselves as specialists as they built departments and established teaching clinics. Beginning in the 1880s, brief periods of intensive training in one of the new post-graduate medical schools in New York and other metropolitan centers allowed established general practitioners to formally acquire specialized knowledge and skills.[3]

John Shaw Billings, best known for compiling the *Index-Catalogue of the Library of the Surgeon General's Office* and something of an expert on the American medical scene, took a slightly sour view of the new medical specialists:

> We have in our cities, great and small, a much larger class of physicians whose principal object is to obtain money, or rather

---

[1] Ira Rutkow, *American Surgery: An Illustrated History* (Philadelphia: Lippincott-Raven, 1998), 174.

[2] For an analysis of specialization in the late-nineteenth century, see: William G. Rothstein, *American Physicians in the Nineteenth Century: From Sects to Science* (Baltimore: Johns Hopkins University Press, 1985), 198-216.

[3] For a history of the post-graduate medical schools in New York and Philadelphia, see Steven J. Peitzman, "'Thoroughly Practical': America's Polyclinic Medical Schools," *Bulletin of the History of Medicine* 54 (1980): 166-87.

the social position, pleasures, and power, which money only can bestow. They are clear-headed, shrewd, practical men, well-educated, because "it pays," and for the same reason they take good care to be supplied with the best instruments, and the latest literature. Many of them take up specialties because the work is easier, and the hours of labour are more under their control than in general practice. They strive to become connected with hospitals and medical schools, not for the love of mental exertion, or of science for its own sake, but as a respectable means of advertising, and of obtaining consultation. They write and lecture to keep their names before the public, and they must do both well, or fall behind in the race. They have the greater part of the valuable practice, and their writings, which constitute the greater part of our medical literature, are respectable in quality and eminently useful.[4]

It seemed as if there would soon be no organs or diseases left for the general practitioner! Townsend reprinted a wry observation by Abraham Jacobi, a distinguished and influential New York physician (and himself one of America's first specialists in the diseases of children), on the subject of specialization:

The general practitioner will in future obtain as the legitimate province of his practice, the male half of mankind, and very old women, and very young children, provided he will keep his hands off their eyes, ears, nervous system, lungs, heart, urinary organs, venereal diseases, nose, pharynx, larynx, skin, hair, and corns.[5]

A contributor to *The Country Practitioner*, mysteriously signing himself "Watson," shared Jacobi's low opinion of the "mere specialist, since many of them get to be hobbyists and seem to

---

4   John Shaw Billings, "Literature and Institutions," in Edward H. Clarke, Henry J. Bigelow, Samuel D. Gross, T. Gaillard Thomas, J.S. Billings, *A Century of American Medicine 1776-1876* (Philadelphia: Henry C. Lea, 1876; repr. New York: Burt Franklin, 1971), 363-64.

5   Abraham Jacobi, "Dr. A. Jacobi Says," *CP* 2, no. 9 (February 1881): 318; reprinted from *New York Medical Record*, no further citation.

think everything comes up under their domain." During "Watson's" forty years in general practice (the location of his practice was not mentioned), he had "known specialists to come to the country and make mistakes of diagnosis which would be a disgrace to an intelligent country physician sufficient to destroy his practice."[6]

Particularly irritating were the patients who demanded referral to a specialist even when the general practitioner felt he had the situation well in hand. Townsend, for example, at the insistence of the patient's husband, accompanied a woman with "a functional affection of the heart" to the office of a well-known Philadelphia surgeon, one of Townsend's former medical school professors. The professor examined the woman in a cursory fashion, confirmed Townsend's prescriptions and added a few of his own as a "mental placebo." A second woman under Townsend's care for neurasthenia and intestinal complaints insisted that a specialist be called in to examine her for anal fissures. The surgeon came, performed an unnecessary minor surgical procedure, collected his fee of one hundred dollars, and left Townsend to deal with a prolonged convalescence. Clearly, Townsend was not dazzled by these particular consultants, whatever the patients may have thought. He concluded that patients should trust their family physician to seek appropriate consultation when indicated.[7]

Despite the pitfalls of country practice, recent medical school graduates, it seems, often found it even harder going in the city, where specialists tended to take over interesting cases. According to an article reprinted in the *Country Practitioner* from the *Pacific Medical and Surgical Reporter* on the subject of country versus city practice, building a practice was easier in the countryside and might take as little as two to three years, compared to five to ten years in the city.[8]

Townsend and like-minded New Jersey colleagues were not alone in their distrust of specialists. Initially, in the 1850s and 1860s, general practitioners, who worked arduous days and nights for at best a modest income, opposed specialization on the grounds

---

6   Watson, "Leaves from the Diary of a Country Doctor," *CP* 2, no. 11 (April 1881): 363.

7   [EPT], "City and Country Doctors," *CP* 1, no. 8 (January 1880): 258-61.

8   "Country versus City Practice" *CP* 1, no. 3 (August 1879): 134-35; reprinted from *Pacific Medical and Surgical Reporter*, no further citation.

that narrowing the field of practice subverted the time-honored medical traditions of the experienced general practitioner, the model of the complete physician. Leading Philadelphia surgeon Samuel D. Gross saw specialization as a negative trend in American medicine:

> In short, American men are general practitioners, ready for the most part, if well educated, to meet any and every emergency, whether in medicine, surgery, or midwifery. Of late, the specialists have seriously encroached upon the province of the general practitioner, and, while they are undoubtedly doing much good, it is questionable whether the arrangement is not also productive of much harm. The soundest, and, therefore, the safest, practitioner is, by all odds, the general practitioner, provided he is thoroughly educated, and fully up to his work.[9]

No doubt, general practitioners also saw unfair competition for scarce patient dollars and the threat of what is now known as "cherry picking," in which choice (i.e., paying or, today, well-insured) patients would gravitate to an array of well-regarded specialists, leaving generalists with the chronically ill and those too poor to travel to urban centers or pay the fees of specialists. Perhaps troublesome patients might return to the general practitioner after the specialist lost interest in the case, or, as in Townsend's example, the generalist might be left to supervise a long convalescence after an ill-advised surgical procedure.

New Jersey practitioners devoted considerable thought to the medical specialists and the rapid expansion of medical knowledge. J. Henry Clark, the historian of the Essex District Medical Society, spoke of a "golden age of medicine all about us," and sympathized with the older practitioner who could no longer absorb or master the expanding range of information and skills. He stressed the Janus-like essence of medicine as both an art and a science, adhering to an honorable ancient tradition as

---

[9]   Samuel D. Gross, "Surgery," in Clarke, et al., *A Century of American Medicine 1776-1876*, 118.

well as the new scientific medicine. He hinted at the difficulties of general practice and the rise of the still unstructured medical specialties: "If you cannot be eminent in every department of medical science, in this day of wonderful expansion, till it seems to cover all the physical sciences, determine to fathom *some well of truth—to feel bottom somewhere.*" The next half century, Clark told his Newark colleagues, "will advance us quite as rapidly and as far as has the last. It depends on us whether we be in the foreground of medical investigation and progress, or be reported among the stragglers."[10] The specialists were here to stay, whether they were New Jersey men or consultants called in from New York and Philadelphia.

Why did Townsend, with his sound education and broad interests, not pursue specialty training when it became available in short courses open to graduate physicians in the decades after the Civil War? Such courses, which relied heavily on the "clinical material" in urban dispensaries and hospitals, were offered for a fee by post-graduate medical schools located in urban centers such as New York and Philadelphia. The sheer necessity of making a living was no doubt Townsend's first priority in the mid-1860s and there was no viable alternative to general practice at that time. Townsend, judging from the pages of the *Country Practitioner*, liked being a generalist. He was confident that the generalist who took the pains to keep abreast of the medical literature could manage the vast majority of illnesses. The near impossibility of succeeding in the competitive environments of New York and Philadelphia at mid-career, together with his family obligations, were further barriers to specialization. For many who did identify themselves as specialists, general practice continued to occupy much of their time. With Townsend's late-career move to the Montana frontier in the 1890s, any thought of specialization vanished.

In general, Townsend's journal was aimed at the established practitioner rather than the man starting out. He recognized that there were discontents in both city and country practice. In his tenth issue, he published a brief and rather anecdotal article

---

[10] J. Henry Clark, "The First Fifty Years of the District Medical Society of Essex County," *TMSNJ* (1867): 177-78, italics in original.

received from a Philadelphia physician who contrasted city and country practice. The city doctor enjoyed the opportunity to look in more often on difficult cases and to respond quickly to a sudden change in the patient's condition. He enjoyed the security of knowing that specialists and colleagues were near at hand and could, if he wished, decline obstetrical, gynecological, or surgical cases. Yet, the country practitioner who had a "frequent longing for a city practice" should know that many country doctors "had left their comfortable homesteads, unexpectedly, to live out the remaining years of their life in poverty and misery" in the city where a "lucrative business must be done to enable a city practitioner to live in style . . . ." Furthermore, riding on cobblestoned streets and "tramping" on pavement were as hard on a weary city man called out in the middle of the night as the "long and tiresome journeys over rough and hilly roads, storms and midnight darkness" so familiar to his country colleague.[11]

Most of Townsend's concerns, however, were for the care of the patient. The country doctor often had to rely on the ability of his patients and their families to follow directions between visits as partners in their own care. While he expected compliance with his medical orders, he appreciated that some families required instruction in the most basic of nursing procedures:

> Every country practitioner should be an accomplished cook and able to go to the kitchen and preparer any dish he may desire for his patient. I have frequently performed such duties and had the satisfaction of seeing my convalescent patients enjoy the dishes that had before been refused with disgust.[12]

The "Domestic Department" of the journal, an ongoing series of practical guides to be shared with patients, covered such issues as home remedies, household perils, rules for the care of the eyes, quack remedies, and popular fallacies. Regarding popular fallacies, Townsend wrote that one of the "most arduous duties of the physician is that of combating false opinions among the

---

[11] S.S. Stauffer, "The Country Medical Practitioner in Contrast with the City Practitioner," *CP* 1, no. 10 (March 1880): 334, 335.

[12] [EPT], "Diet for the Sick," *CP* 2, no. 6 (November 1880): 193.

people, that have descended from generation to generation." Among the popular fallacies addressed were a strong belief in the value of sea-bathing (often overdone) and the failure to recognized that summer diarrhea in children was often due to faulty feeding practices with subsequent decomposition and "catarrh of the digestive tract."[13]

. There were also proto-psychology articles such as "Sleeplessness from Thought."[14] Townsend seems to have been a kind-hearted man, sympathetic to the plight of hard-working country and village women. He included at least two articles on practical psychology in the "Domestic Department." From *Sanitary Magazine*, he borrowed "Weary Woman," a short piece which attributed weariness to overwork. The solution was simple: "for the sake of humanity, let the work go." It was better, continued the unknown author, "to live in the midst of disorder than that order should be purchased at so high a price—the cost of health, strength, happiness, and all that makes existence endurable."[15] Some of his readers and most farm and village husbands of the time would have considered this a radical notion indeed. In a second article, borrowed from *Good Health*, the issue of "Why Women Fade" was taken up. Briefly, the culprits were improper rest, drudgery, fretfulness, and want of fresh air.[16]

Diseases of the mind attracted much attention at the time. The superintendent of Sunnyside Medical Retreat (New York) for Mental and Nervous Disorders contributed an article on "Mental Responsibility and the Diagnosis of Insanity in Criminal Cases."[17]

---

[13] [EPT], "Domestic Department: Popular Fallacies," *CP* 2, no. 8 (January 1881): 262; "Household Perils," "Sea-Bathing," Summer Diarrhoeas of Children," 263-5. Notes on sea-bathing and infantile diarrhea reprinted from *Good Health*, no further citation. Today we would attribute such seasonal diarrhea in children either to viral or bacterial gastroenteritis. Poor hygiene, unsafe water and milk, and inadequate refrigeration and food handling were the major contributory factors.

[14] "Domestic Department: Sleeplessness from Thought," *CP* 2, no. 12 (May 1881): 402-4; reprinted from Grandville, "Common Mind Troubles," no further citation.

[15] "Domestic Department: Weary Women," *CP* 2, no. 12 (May 1881): 404; reprinted from *Sanitary Magazine*, no further citation.

[16] "Domestic Department: Why Women Fade," *CP* 3, no. 1 (July 1881): 14-16; reprinted from *Good Health*, no further citation.

[17] Edward C. Mann, "Mental Responsibility and the Diagnosis of Insanity in Criminal Cases," *CP*, no. 2 (July, 1879): 10-20.

The management of neurasthenia and hysteria, both high-profile and modish abnormalities of psyche and soma, were the subject of an essay by the acknowledged American authority in the field, Dr. S. Weir Mitchell of Philadelphia."[18]

Townsend did not shrink from the mundane. An editorial plea for public toilets framed the issue in terms of public health: "Every physician knows that a great number of the physical ailments of mankind—male and female—are produced by inattention to these calls [of nature] . . . ."[19] Whether a matter of health or convenience, the problem of public toilets remains unsolved long after the publication of Townsend's brief editorial.

The opportunity to air his well-considered views and the slight prestige that the *Country Practitioner* brought him were Townsend's humble rewards. Perhaps John Shaw Billings had been correct in pointing out that no amount of sensible advice could discourage a man from founding a medical journal. Townsend would soon come to agree with that observation. He was correct in identifying an underserved readership of country practitioners across America, and seemed truly disappointed by what he perceived to be ungrateful potential subscribers and indifferent potential contributors.

---

[18]   S. Weir Mitchell, "Neurasthenia, Hysteria, and Their Treatment," *CP* 2, no. 1 (July 1879): 19-22; reprinted from *Chicago Medical Gazette*, no further citation. Mitchell is best remembered for devising the "rest cure" for neurasthenia.

[19]   [EPT], "Public Accommodations," *CP* 1, no. 11 (April 1880): 398.

CHAPTER 10

AN EDITOR'S WOES

Editing and publishing a small monthly medical journal was a merciless task under any circumstances, but even more so when the editor, publisher, and circulation manager were all embodied in the same active general practitioner. Most such journals disappeared quickly. Like other medical publishers and editors, Townsend suffered from a chronic dearth of contributions. Many issues were padded with borrowed articles and editorial commentaries by Townsend. In the course of the two-year life of the *Country Practitioner*, Townsend resorted to a variety of techniques from suggestion to flattery to chastisement, to encourage his readers to contribute articles.

In the first issue of the *Country Practitioner*, Townsend led off with an obstetric metaphor: "Having gone safely through the pangs of labor, it will depend, gentlemen, upon the kind of pabulum you furnish in our infancy whether we survive, or perish from—*marasmus* [severe malnutrition]."[1] Hoping to whip up enthusiasm among potential contributors, he gently lambasted his subscribers in the third issue, noting that only one in three hundred physicians communicates with a medical journal:

> Do you believe you have any right to practice medicine for
> a lifetime, gain a fund of valuable experience, die, and leave

---

[1]   Ellis P. Townsend, "To Medical Practitioners," *CP* 1, no. 1 (June 1879): 3.

your family nothing but a worn out medicine case, your obstetric forceps, and a rusty old pocket case [surgical kit] by which to prove your usefulness in the profession? Or shall they point with pride to the record of your good works, as given in your communications to a "medical journal."

Appealing to the pride of New Jersey physicians, he added:

We are trying to give New Jersey one [medical journal], because we believe that New Jersey physicians are doing as good work as any others, and know that they have plenty of experience that should be recorded . . . . Our columns are at the disposal of County Societies and physicians from Maine to Texas, and from the Atlantic to the Pacific.[2]

Townsend went so far as to badger his ailing and aged father for a contribution. W.W. Townsend of Bridesburg, Pennsylania, responded to his son's insistence that he give "so much of his experience as his enfeebled health and impaired eyesight will permit." The elder Townsend's subject was the use of propylamine chloride in acute inflammatory rheumatism, a treatment that he had used with success for a quarter of a century.[3]

Townsend took up his restless editorial pen again in the sixth issue to prod his reluctant country brethren to make some account of themselves by contributing to his journal. The poor reputation that country doctors enjoyed among their city brethren was inevitable judging "by the small additions many country doctors make to the medical literature of the day . . . Unfortunately the majority of [county doctors] have as great a dread of pen and ink as a rabid dog for water . . . ." On the contrary, maintained Townsend, the country "is full of intelligent, hard working, successful practitioners," who must hone their skills carefully, lest an untimely obstetrical or surgical death destroy reputations always at the mercy of wagging country tongues. Helpfully, he

---

[2] Ellis P. Townsend, "Editorial," *CP* 1, no. 3 (August 1879): 106.
[3] W.W. Townsend, "Propylamine Chloride in Acute Inflammatory Rheumatism," *CP* 1, no. 5 (October 1879): 147.

pointed out that the long winter evenings were a "good time for those who are accustomed to writing to send in a little of their work." For novice writers, it was a good time to "cultivate the habit."[4]

In the final issue of the first year, Townsend attempted to inspire his readers to contribute to his journal by praising their skills and boosting their self-confidence. They need have no fear," he wrote, of "the criticism or sneers from the (so-called) high authorities" when submitting articles. Townsend maintained that he was "fully satisfied after a year's examination of half a hundred exchanges, that fully as much nonsense is promulgated by the said high authorities as by the lesser lights."[5] Halfway through the second year of publication, he tried a new tactic: "Gentlemen," he intoned in an editorial, "we have waited patiently for you to get through with your annual vacations, and must now ask you to report what you are doing among your cases."[6]

A new feature in the second year of publication was "Leaves from the Diaries" of country practitioners; the emphasis was on isolation in country practice and submissions were solicited from readers:

> The object is to record difficult and troublesome cases, hundreds of which occur in the practice of every isolated physician, and frequently from the want of instruments and appliances, and in the absence of assistance[,] success is accomplished if at all, by means that would seem inadequate . . . . Our object in asking these reports and publishing them is that they may suggest expedients to the young practitioner in similar emergencies.[7]

By the sixth issue of the second volume, Townsend was appealing for subscribers as well as contributors: "There is not a country doctor in New Jersey or any other State worthy of the title

---

4   [EPT], "Editorial," *CP* 1, no. 6 (November 1879): 213-15.
5   [EPT], "Editorial", *CP* 1, no. 12 (May 1880): 435.
6   EPT, "Our Subscribers," *CP* 2, no. 3 (August 1880): 105.
7   [EPT], "Editorial," *CP* 2, no. 11 (April 1881): 388-89.

he claims, who cannot afford to invest two dollars, to support the only journal that advocates his interests exclusively . . . . [8]

At the end of two years, he asked editorially "*Qui-bono?*" [sic]—to whose benefit? "Personally it has been a source of constant labor, but a labor that is in accordance with our tastes . . . . The editor is himself a hard-working country practitioner who has been under fire for eighteen years and hence more practical than theoretic in his views."[9]

Despite the irritating lack of contributors and readers, Townsend's spirits were buoyed at the half-year point by "many letters of commendation and encouragement from all parts of the country . . . ."[10] Commenting on the first issue, a writer from Danville, Kentucky congratulated Townsend on his "chaste and manly salutatory." In something of a *non sequitur,* the correspondent took the opportunity to remind Townsend that country doctor Ephraim McDowell of Danville, operating on a table in his home, had pioneered abdominal surgery by successfully removing a giant ovarian cyst from a country woman in 1809.[11] A year later, Townsend was pleased to quote the *Therapeutic Gazette:* "The snap with which Dr. Townsend permeates his little journal makes the paper very readable . . . ."[12] Townsend noted with pride that "[q]uite a number of the leading physicians of Philadelphia are subscribers and speak well of the journal."[13] In the same issue, however, came a tart response to the editor of the *American Bi-Weekly,* who "estimates the value of our journal at forty-one cents." "Thank you brother," added Townsend, "we were uncertain as to its value."[14]

Much can be learned about the state of medical practice from advertisements. For Townsend, who urged his readers to patronize the advertisers, the half and full-page advertisements ($10 and $15 respectively) were a welcome source of revenue. Frequent

---

8   [EPT], "Personal," *CP* 2, no. 6, (November 1880): 211.
9   [EPT], "Editorial," *CP* 2, no. 12 (May 1881): 423.
10   [EPT], "Editorial," *CP* 1, no. 7 (December 1879): 251.
11   S.Q. Lapian, "Letter to the Editor," *CP* 1, no. 3 (August 1879): 87.
12   [EPT], "Editorial," *CP* 2, no. 7 (December 1880): 248.
13   [EPT], "Editorial," *CP* 2, no.10 (March 1881): 353.
14   [EPT], "Editorial," *CP* 2, no. 10 (March 1881): 354.

advertisers included medical/surgical instrument suppliers such as S.S. Staufer ("hard rubber uterine instruments") and Horatio G. Kern ("surgical and dental instruments, trusses, etc."). Pharmaceutical advertisements included Keasby and Mattison's Dextro Quinine (an anti-malaria preparation), Powell's Combined Beef, Cod-Liver Oil and Pepsin ("a general nutriment and Tonic invigorator"), Battle and Co.'s Bromidia ("the hypnotic par excellence"), Parke-Davis' Hoang-Nan (a strychnine preparation), Coca ("a nervous stimulant of very decided activity"), and Jamaica Dogwood ("a substitute for opium in many painful afflictions"). The Sunnyside Medical Retreat for Mental and Nervous Diseases, Inebriety, and the Opium Habit took out a quarter-page advertisement. Bellevue Hospital Medical College and the University of the City of New York Medical Department took out full-page advertisements detailing faculty, fees, course of study, and attractive educational features such as dissecting rooms and access to hospital clinics.

Townsend was mortified when he was compelled to confess to his readers that he had lost a submitted article:

> We were unfortunate enough to mislay or lose a valuable article on the "Therapy of Veratrum Viridi" [sic] by one of our most esteemed correspondents. We especially regret this, as it was an article of great importance, on a medicine that very few practitioners know the value of. It is needless to say such carelessness shall not be repeated.[15]

With the third issue of the third volume, published in September 1881, the *Country Practitioner*, with no word of explanation, ceased publication.[16] Townsend had clearly expected at the time to continue publication, for he included a request for information from readers about their experience with vaccination for smallpox. His intention was to prepare a statistical report on current vaccination practices. His detailed questionnaire was

---

[15]   [EPT], "Editorial," *CP* 2, no. 8 (January 1881): 285.
[16]   Volume 2, no. 12 was issued in May 1881. Apologizing for being "in the lurch," Townsend did not issue volume 3, no. 1 until July, 1881; [EPT], "Editorial,", *CP* 3, no. 1 (July 1881): 39.

printed in the final issue and he anticipated that all who replied to the questionnaire would receive a copy of the report.[17]

The immediate cause of the decision to close the *Country Practitioner* may have been ill health in the family, although this is only speculation. According to the 1880 census, Townsend's wife, Almira "Jennie" Johnston Townsend, bore four living children and three other children known to have died in early childhood or infancy. Almira's older sister, listed in the census as a "servant," had been living with the Townsend family from as early as 1870.[18] It is possible that Mrs. Townsend suffered from chronic ill health and required her husband's time and attention in addition to her sister's assistance, making it impossible for him to devote the necessary hours to his journal in addition to the demands of practice. Although the nature of Townsend's wife's illness is unknown, the most common fatal illness at that time among young adults would have been tuberculosis. Family lore (unconfirmed) suggests that she indeed suffered from consumption.[19]

After the *Country Practitioner* ceased publication, Townsend continued to practice in Beverly for another year. His name remained on the rolls of the Burlington County Medical Society through 1882 and appeared again as an "honorary member" in 1886.[20] In 1883, the country practitioner moved on to the nearby city of Camden, New Jersey.

---

[17] [EPT], "Notes and Comments: Vaccination," *CP* 3, no. 3 (September 1881): 86-87; "Editorial (smallpox, followed by questionnaire," *CP* 3, no. 3 (September 1881): 116-18.

[18] 1880 census accessed through Ancestry.com which includes scans of original census enumerators' worksheets, http://renesfamily.com/family/family. php?famid=F00439&ged=Renes.ged. Documented genealogical research courtesy René Delaney's website at http://renesfamily.com/family/individual. php?pid=I01010&ged=Renes.GED and personal communication. Children: Oscar (b. 1862, d. 1865), William W. (b. 1864, d. 1888 in York, PA), Eleanor (b. 1866, d. 1869), Charles M. (b. 1868, d. 1894 in Billings MT), John P. (b. 1871, d. 1906 in Frankford PA of Brights disease [kidney failure] and buried Beverly NJ), Alice B. (b. 1876, d. 1944, history unknown), Edith G. (b?, d. 7 months). Mary Johnston, Almira's sister, was two years older than Almira; she was listed in the 1870 and 1880 census lists, with the designation "servant" in the 1880 list.

[19] Personal communication, René Delaney.

[20] "Members of District Medical Societies: Burlington County," *TMSNJ* (1882), 10; *TMSNJ* (1886), 10.

CHAPTER 11

MEDICAL LIFE IN THE BIG(GER) CITY

Townsend left Beverly for Camden, (Camden County), New Jersey, some fifteen miles down the Delaware River from Beverly and directly across the river from Philadelphia, in late 1882 or 1883.[1] At a regular meeting of the Burlington County Medical Society in April, 1883, Townsend "tendered his resignation as an active member which was accepted, he having moved out of the county." Townsend was present at this meeting and, as usual, participated in the discussions of medical cases.[2] The reasons for Townsend's move to Camden are unknown. His income may have been insufficient or, perhaps, he found the small town too confining. There is no hint of professional conflict, but the secretary of the county medical society might have purposely omitted such details from the minute book.

---

[1] John R. Stevenson, "A History of Medicine and Medical Men," in *A History of the Camden County Medical and Surgical Society*, ed. George R. Prowell (Philadelphia: L.J. Richards, 1886), 294. Stevenson gives September, 1884, as the date of Townsend's arrival in Camden. The exact date of his departure from Burlington is unknown. There may have been a few months of professional inactivity as he relocated his family and his practice.

[2] *Burlington County Medical Society Minute Book: 1869-1893* (entry April 10, 1883).

If, indeed, Townsend's wife suffered from tuberculosis during the last months or years in Beverly, the move to Camden might have been on her account. Perhaps Townsend sought more expert medical advice for his wife or a more remunerative practice to provide for her nursing or sanitarium care. It is possible, though less likely, that her death at age forty-four in Camden in January, 1884, followed complications of a late pregnancy or other acute illness unrelated to tuberculosis.[3]

Camden, with close to forty-two thousand residents, was ranked forty-fourth in population among American cities in 1880.[4] The medical community was strong and thriving, with long-standing ties to the medical colleges and leading physicians of Philadelphia. Like Townsend, many Camden practitioners had trained at one of the Philadelphia medical schools. In 1883, a tabulation by the Camden County (or District) Medical Society of close to nine hundred deaths gives an indication of the type of serious cases a general practitioner like Townsend might be expected to see. Most deaths were ascribed to tuberculosis (phthisis pulmonalis) and a variety of infections such as pneumonia, scarlet fever, typhoid, diphtheria, and undifferentiated infantile diarrhea (cholera infantum).[5]

Camden was sufficiently large to warrant a city medical society, but the organization had struggled with failing membership and intermittent suspensions of meetings over the years. In 1883, Townsend was elected to membership in the Camden City Medical Society. It was a sign of the organization's weakness that Townsend was elected vice-president at the same time he was inducted into the society. The following year (1884), he was elected president. His paper on "Modern Therapeutics" was one of just two presentations for that year. In 1889, he gave a

---

[3]   The death of Almira Johnston, which occurred in Camden, N.J. on January 5th, 1883 was recorded in the *Burlington Gazette*, 12 January 1884, p. 3; courtesy René Delaney.

[4]   United States Bureau of the Census, "Population of the 100 Largest Urban Places: 1880," http://www.census.gov/population/www/documentation/twps0027/tab11.txt (accessed July 31, 2010).

[5]   Jno. W. Snowden, "Reports of District Societies: Camden County," *TMSNJ* (1884): 195.

paper on uterine hemorrhage, reflecting his ongoing interest in obstetrics and gynecology. He was not mentioned among the officers or committee members of the city medical society in 1885 or 1886, but was again active as a member of the by-laws and constitution committee in 1887. In 1889 through 1892, he was named a representative of the Camden City Medical Society to the managing board of the Camden City Dispensary. For a number of years, he directed the ophthalmology clinic at the dispensary and continued this volunteer service after the clinic was expanded to include both eye and ear diseases in 1892. Such service usually required a few hours or a half day weekly.[6]

Booster that he was, Townsend was pleased to inform the county society in 1888 that his little city medical society ("despite ups and downs" for several decades) was enjoying "remarkable success" and had "succeeded in uniting the medical men of the city more closely to their common interest."[7] A new professional organization, the Camden City Medical and Surgical Society, appeared on the scene in November, 1891. It is unclear whether this was a new society or the successor to the Camden City Medical Society. In any case, Townsend was elected the first president. The ambitious mission of the society was to hear monthly reports on medicine, surgery, pathology, chemistry, therapeutics, hygiene, and dietetics. Townsend either resigned from membership or was not reelected to any office in 1892.[8]

In contrast to Camden's city medical societies, the Camden Country Medical Society was strong and well-organized, with forty-six members as of 1887. Its meetings were marked by vigorous discussion and useful papers. Guest speakers such as the prominent William Pepper, M.D., of Philadelphia, a professor of medicine at the University of Pennsylvania, added to the educational value of the meetings.[9] At a meeting of the

6   E.L.B. Godfrey, *History of the Medical Profession of Camden County, New Jersey* (Camden: F.A. Davis, 1896), 154, 186, 228-30, 233.

7   EPT, "Reports of District Societies: Camden County," *TMSNJ* (1888): 187.

8   Godfrey, *History of the Medical Profession of Camden County*, 279.

9   Godfrey, *History of the Medical Profession of Camden County*, 193; "Members of District Medical Societies," *TMSNJ* (1887): 10-11.

county society in November, 1883, Townsend was elected to membership.[10] His name first appeared on the published rolls of the society in 1884, but he was not listed as a member between 1885 and 1886.[11] Taking into account the fact that rosters were published only once yearly, it is safe to say that he was absent from Camden, or at least absent from the county society, in 1884 and 1885. An obituary published at the time of his death in 1907 by a newspaper in Billings, Montana, commented that Townsend had practiced for a number of years in Philadelphia and worked at a government pension office in Washington before coming to Billings.[12] Although neither statement could be confirmed, it is entirely possible that he worked in Philadelphia and/or Washington during these two years of apparent absence from Camden.

Townsend's name reappeared in minutes of the Camden County Medical Society in late 1886, when he was appointed to a committee to investigate the water supplies in towns and cities across Camden County.[13] His interest in this public health issue continued for several years; he pointed out in 1889 that the water supply of the city of Camden had deteriorated.[14] In 1887, when his name reappeared on the annual membership lists, he informed the society that his practice in the last year had "little of general interest," except for rather virulent epidemics of measles and chicken pox. His crusade against the misdiagnosis and mistreatment of diphtheria, begun in Burlington County and continued through the pages of the *Country Practitioner*, was reactivated by a fatal case in his Camden practice. The symptoms, probably in a child, included "[p]aralysis of the muscles of deglutition [swallowing], hemorrhage from throat and nares [nostrils], paralysis of heart . . . . death completed the work on the eighth day." He once again chided those who attributed cures to useless remedies and claimed they had never lost a case.[15]

---

10 Godfrey, *History of the Medical Profession of Camden County,* 54, 156, 189-91.
11 Members of District Medical Societies," *TMSNJ* (1884): 10; (1885): 10; (1886): 10.
12 "Dr. Townsend Answers Call: Death Summons Well Known Billings Physician," *Billings Daily Gazette,* July 31, 1907.
13 Godfrey, *History of the Medical Profession of Camden County,* 194.
14 EPT, "Reports of District Societies: Camden County," *TMSNJ* (1889): 187-89.
15 "Members of District Medical Societies," *TMSNJ* (1887): 10-11; John W. Snowden, "Reports of District Societies: Camden County," *TMSNJ* (1887): 312-13.

Although he was not directly involved in the building or staffing of Camden's Cooper Hospital, Townsend reported to the state medical society in 1889 that the hospital, a private charitable venture, was open and receiving patients. Medical and surgical facilities were excellent: "For convenience, appliances and equipment, it has no superior in this country." Some fifty patients in wards or private rooms were attended by eight private Camden physicians and surgeons, as well as two house doctors and a pathologist.[16] Townsend certainly knew the members of the hospital's medical staff and may have had occasion to refer patients to the hospital from time to time.

With the opening of the Cooper Hospital, Camden was beginning a transition to hospital-based medical and surgical care that reflected national trends. Cooper was not however, Camden's first hospital; the West Jersey Hospital had opened there in 1885 under the direction of homeopathic physicians. The old tensions between homeopaths and regulars were beginning to fade, and the homeopaths (and eclectics) were increasingly being accepted as part of the legitimate medical brotherhood. When New Jersey finally formed a state board of medical examiners in 1890, it was mandated that five members be regulars, three homeopaths, and one eclectic. The Medical Society of New Jersey would have preferred two boards—one for the regulars and one for sectarians, but the legislature did not agree.[17]

Townsend had maintained in the pages of the *Country Practitioner*, that motivated country physicians could capably manage most of their cases and that, with some exceptions, big-city specialists were rarely needed.[18] Now that he was an urban physician in a mid-sized community, Townsend continued to celebrate local medical talent. He was pleased to note in 1888, for example, that well-trained consultants, some specializing in surgery, were available right in Camden: "Fewer visits have

---

[16] EPT, "Reports of District Societies: Camden County," *TMSNJ* (1888): 185.

[17] David L. Cowen, *Medicine and Health in New Jersey: A History* (Princeton: D. Van Nostrand, 1964), 74, 127. New threats from osteopathy, chiropractic, and optometry ensured that the battle for legitimacy would continue.

[18] For example, see [EPT], "City and Country Doctors," *CP* 1, no. 8 (January 1880): 258-61.

been made in Camden by Philadelphia consulting physicians and surgeons during the past year than at any time formerly. It has been discovered that there are men on this side [i.e. the New Jersey side of the Delaware River] who can make a diagnosis, open a trachea, or even remove an offending uterus, as well as irritating ovaries, successfully."[19]

New Jersey's county and state medical societies regularly elected standing committees or "reporters." Instituted in 1820, such committees were charged with investigating and reporting "the general state of health of the citizens of New Jersey, during the preceding year, the causes, nature and cure of the epidemics (if any have prevailed) in any part of the State, curious medical facts and discoveries, and remarkable cases that may have come to their knowledge."[20] Over the decades, reporters for the county and state societies were generally the more scientifically engaged members. These reports of county and state standing committees formed the scientific backbone of the *Transactions of the Medical Society of New Jersey*, and were, in effect, longitudinal narratives of the professional activities of physicians and the prevailing health conditions across the state in the decades before organized public health reporting.

At the 1887 meeting of the Camden County Medical Society, Townsend was elected chairman of the standing committee, a decided honor for such a new member of the Camden medical community. (The title of "reporter" was used in the membership roster, although minutes of the meeting referred to "standing committee.") Townsend was re-elected to the post from 1888 through 1892.[21] In his capacity as reporter, he attended the statewide

---

19   EPT, "Reports of District Societies: Camden County," *TMSNJ* (1888): 187.

20   Stephen Wickes, ed., *The Rise, Minutes, and Proceedings of the New Jersey Medical Society, Established July 23rd, 1766* (Newark: Jennings and Hardham, 1875), 188.

21   Godfrey, *History of the Medical Profession of Camden County*, 194, 196, 238, 239, 240. Townsend's name again disappears from the published roster of the society in 1889, although his report on Camden County activities is included in the minutes; "Members of District Societies," *TMSNJ* (1889), 10-1; EPT, "Reports of District Societies: Camden County," *TMSNJ* (1889): 183-89.

meeting of the Medical Society of New Jersey in 1889.[22] As a former editor, the post of reporter would have been quite congenial to Townsend, involving as it did the gathering, analysis, editing, and reporting of clinical and epidemiological information. Reporters for the various county societies had long complained about the paucity of information provided by rank and file members to the reporter, a state of affairs familiar to Townsend from his years as editor of the *Country Practitioner*.

There is some confusion about Townsend's whereabouts in 1889 and 1890. It is possible that he was practicing in Philadelphia while continuing to attend meetings of the Camden County Medical Society. In 1889 and again in 1890, he was not listed as a member of the Camden County Medical Society in the annual *Transactions of the Medical Society of New Jersey*. However, he was mentioned in the minutes and submitted his annual report in 1889. It appears as if Townsend was either absent from Camden for months at a time or the rosters were incorrectly drawn up. His report on the medical status of Camden County for 1889 was submitted and printed in the same volume of the *Transactions*.[23] At the 1890 meeting of the Medical Society of New Jersey, and again in 1891, Townsend was elected a member of the state standing committee, a post of considerable responsibility.[24] The standing committee of two or three members was responsible for compiling annual reports on local health conditions submitted by the county medical societies.

In 1889, Townsend was one of three Camden physicians appointed to the United States Pension Board of Examining Surgeons, a post he held until 1892. Almost three decades after Appomattox, military pension claims were a growing concern. The medical pension board was established in Camden in 1884

[22]   William Pierson, "Transactions of the Medical Society of New Jersey: The One Hundred and Twenty-Third Annual Meeting," *TMSNJ* (1889): 25.

[23]   "Members of District Societies," *TMSNJ* (1889): 10-11, *TMSNJ* (1890): 10-11; EPT, "Reports of District Societies: Camden County," *TMSNJ* (1889): 183-9; Godfrey, *History of the Medical Profession of Camden County*, 197, 237-8.

[24]   William Pierson, "Transactions of the Medical Society of New Jersey: The One Hundred and Twenty-Fourth Annual Meeting," *TMSNJ* (1890): 73; William Pierson, "Transactions of the Medical Society of New Jersey: The One Hundred and Twenty-Fifth Annual Meeting," *TMSNJ* (1891): 50.

with the purpose of examining applicants locally for veterans' benefits.[25]

Officially back on the roster of the Camden County Medical Society in 1891, Townsend's report on members' medical activities and the state of the county's health for that year included a familiar refrain. Adopting the tart and cynical tone he had used from time to time in the *Country Practitioner*, Townsend issued a plea for more contributions of medical news from members: "This year eight members have been courteous enough to reply to my interrogatories, while the rest have presumably consigned them to the waste basket."[26] Lacking input from other members, Townsend used his report to launch a harsh and lengthy criticism of German microbiologist Robert Koch's premature and ill-managed announcement of his discovery of "tuberculin," a purported cure for tuberculosis. Townsend roundly denounced those prominent physicians in Philadelphia and New York (particularly those connected with medical colleges) who had eagerly jumped on the Koch tuberculin bandwagon to the detriment of the profession and their patients. As tuberculin became the target of criticism for its lack of efficacy and dangerous side effects, Koch's American champions were, in Townsend's opinion, "as anxious for the whole episode to be forgotten, as they were crazy to begin it."[27]

Townsend continued as reporter for Camden in 1892, praising the increasingly "self-dependent" surgeons as well as the physicians (i.e., non-surgeons) who were "skillfully reducing the death rate."[28] Clearly, many Camden practitioners had begun to specialize in surgery, while others focused on non-surgical aspects of medical practice. Such distinctions were informal and based mainly local reputation; specialty boards with examining and certification powers were still far in the future. Typical of the concerns of the county society was a discussion of "internal antiseptics" for derangements of the stomach. In their notes to Townsend, Camden physicians variously lauded turpentine,

---

[25]   Godfrey, *History of the Medical Profession of Camden County*, 178.
[26]   EPT, "Reports of District Societies: Camden County," *TMSNJ* (1891): 269.
[27]   Ibid., 272-73.
[28]   EPT, "Reports of District Societies: Camden County," *TMSNJ* (1892): 236.

bismuth sub-iodide, sulpho-carbolate of zinc, creosote, carbolic acid, arsenite of copper, Listerine, and the still-popular mercurial laxatives. All agreed that peritonitis (an inflammation of the lining of the abdomen treated today with broad spectrum antibiotics and surgical intervention when indicated) should be treated with saline cathartics, opium, and external heat.[29]

By 1892, Townsend was on his way up the executive ladder in the Camden County Medical Society. In 1892 and again in 1893, he was elected vice-president, an office that could be expected to lead to the presidency. The society was growing in numbers and prestige within the state; membership by 1893 had increased to fifty-six. In 1890, Dr. Sophia Presley, an 1879 graduate of Woman's Medical College in Philadelphia, became the first "female practitioner of medicine" to be elected to membership in the county medical society, following eight years of rejection.[30] However, within a year of assuming the vice-presidency, Townsend left Camden to begin medical life anew in Billings, Montana. The erstwhile county practitioner was returning to country practice.

---

[29]   Ibid., 237.
[30]   Godfrey, *History of the Medical Profession of Camden County,* 240. "Members of District Medical Societies," *TMSNJ* (1892): 10-11; *TMSNJ* (1893): 10-11, *TMSNJ* (1894): 11; Henry H. Sherk, *Colleagues and Competitors: A Sesquicentennial History of the Camden County Medical Society: 1846-1996* (Voorhees, NJ: Camden County Medical Society, 1996), 81-84.

CHAPTER 12

THE COUNTRY DOCTOR GOES WEST

Townsend's decision to leave Camden appears to have been made rather suddenly. His departure from Camden in 1893 was marked officially by the medical society he had served faithfully for a decade with the brief notation that three members "have removed from the jurisdiction of the Society and have been dropped from the rolls."[1] At the age of fifty-eight, Townsend left for the Big Sky Country of Billings, Montana.

In September, 1886, close to three years after the death of his first wife, Townsend remarried to a much younger woman named Edith Jeannette Sleeper. The Sleeper family, with origins in Ohio and Pennsylvania, had relocated to Burlington City by 1870 from their home in Pennsylvania when Edith was a young child.[2] Burlington was a few miles north of Beverly, and the two cities had social and business ties. It is possible that Townsend knew the Sleeper family while he was still living in Beverly. At the time of her marriage to Townsend, Edith was twenty-five and her husband fifty-one years old.[3] A son, Edward Grubb Townsend, was born to the couple in 1889.[4]

---

[1] Daniel Strock, "Reports of District Societies: Camden County," *TMSNJ* (1893): 209.

[2] 1870 census lists Edith Sleeper, b. 1861, in Burlington, New Jersey.

[3] http://www.renesfamily.com/family/family.php?famid=F00439&ged=Renes.GED.

[4] The name Grubb was undoubtedly chosen in honor of General E. Burd Grubb, a native of Burlington. Townsend mentioned Grubb's nearby estate in his pamphlet,

Townsend's rather unexpected move to Montana was almost certainly related to his ties to the Sleeper family. The *Billings Gazette* noted that Townsend was related by marriage to "a number of prominent Billings people." According to the *Gazette*, Townsend's in-laws in the city included his wife's brother and two married sisters.[5] Census records from 1900 list Joseph Sleeper, a furniture "manager" (it is unclear whether he was a furniture store or furniture factory manager) in Billings, although his date of arrival there is unknown.[6]

It appears that the two eldest sons and a daughter of Townsend's first marriage remained in Pennsylvania with relatives when their father's second family moved west. Both sons died as young men, predeceasing their father. John P., who died of Bright's disease (kidney failure) in 1906 at age thirty-four was a druggist and was buried in Beverly. William W. died in 1888 at age twenty-two in Pennsylvania. Alice B. Townsend, the daughter of Townsend's first marriage, married in 1899 and died in Pennsylvania in 1944. At least one son of Townsend's first marriage, Charles M., (b. 1868), traveled with Ellis and his second family to Billings, where he died in 1894, shortly after arriving in Montana.[7] Edward Grubb Townsend (b. 1899) would have been about five years old when his parents came to Billings; he later worked as superintendent of the Billings power company and died in Billings in 1947 at age fifty-eight.[8] Townsend's last child, daughter, Edith, was born in 1897 in Montana and named for her mother; her father was

---

Suburban Homes. Grubb was a heroic commander of Civil War infantry (twice wounded in ten battles), Burlington industrialist, failed candidate for New Jersey governor, and ambassador to Spain. "General E. Burd Grubb Dies in 72d Year," *New York Times*, July 8, 1913, p. 7.

[5] "Dr. Townsend Answers Call," *Billings Daily Gazette* July 31, 1907, p. 3.

[6] United States census, 1890 and 1900, copies of original census-takers' work sheets, Billings, Montana; accessed through Ancestor.com.

[7] Courtesy René Delaney.

[8] "Funeral Rites Held For Power Official" (Edward Grubb Townsend), *Billings Gazette*, March 26, 1947; photocopy courtesy Montana State Historical Society. Corky Knebel, "T Index for Mountainview Cemetery, Billings, MT.," United States GenWeb Archives, http://files.usgwarchives.org/mt/yellowstone/cemeteries/mtview/t.txt (accessed July 2, 2010). Obituary notice for Edward Grubb Townsend, *Billings Gazette*, n.d.; photocopy courtesy Montana State Historical Society.

sixty-two at the time of her birth.[9] Townsend had his share of sorrow, having outlived his first wife, several infant children, and three adult sons from his first marriage.

Montana Territory, created in 1864, had about twelve thousand residents and perhaps twenty physicians. The region's earliest physicians were associated with exploring expeditions, railroad construction, gold and silver mining, Indian reservations, and army outposts. Montana's medical practitioners belonged to a hardy brotherhood. Journeys of two or three days to remote areas were not unusual. There were no medical societies and little communication. Regular physicians of varying training and ability competed with the usual assortment of sectarians.

Prior to 1880, the Yellowstone Valley, site of the future town of Billings, was Native-American country, mostly Crow Nation. To the south and north there were Cheyenne and some Sioux. The Northern Pacific reached Montana in 1881 and towns advanced westward with the railroad along the Yellowstone River.[10] Townsend arrived in Billings in 1893, just a few years after Montana statehood.[11] The new state was still very much on the American frontier, though statehood marked the beginning of a period of rapid growth.[12] Almost three hundred years after Massachusetts settlers discovered that smallpox had decimated the local Native American tribes, the disease was striking down other Native Americans not far from Billings; when Dr. A.P. Merriweather took over as Crow Agency physician in 1899, he

---

[9]   Census, 1890, original census-taker's work sheets; accessed through Ancestor.com. Townsend and his first wife, Almira, also had a daughter named Edith, who died in infancy. Although it was not uncommon to give subsequent infants the name of a lost child, it is more likely that the daughter of his second marriage was named for her mother.

[10] Paul C. Phillips, *Medicine in the Making of Montana* (Missoula: Montana State University Press, 1962), 378-80.

[11] "Dr. Townsend Answers Call," *Billings Daily Gazette,* July 31, 1907, p. 3; "Obituary: Ellis P. Townsend," *Medical Sentinel* 15 (1907): 454. The *Journal of the American Medical Association*, in its published obituary (1907), recorded Townsend's tenure in Montana as eighteen years, making his date of arrival 1889; "Ellis P. Townsend," Obituary, *Journal of the American Medical Association* 49 (1907): 710. This chronology is incorrect, as Townsend was still active in the Camden County Medical Society in 1891 and 1892.

[12] Phillips, *Medicine in the Making of Montana*, 41-42.

found a smallpox epidemic in progress and vaccinated some two thousand Indians.[13]

Some early residents of Montana were "tuberculars" seeking health in the fresh frontier air, though harsh living conditions probably speeded the deaths of many.[14] It is likely that in Montana, as was the case elsewhere in the American West, consumptive physicians who found their own health improved urged sufferers from back East to come to Montana for healthy air and expert treatment.[15] Dr. L. Rodney Pococke arrived in Helena, Montana, in 1863. According to a historian of western medicine, Pococke came for gold as well as his own health; despite his robust appearance in a photographic portrait, he died of consumption within two years of his arrival.[16]

Billings, located in south central Montana in the Yellowstone Valley, was founded with the coming of the Northern Pacific Railroad in 1877. Dr. Dennis Parker from Vermont established a practice in Billings in 1882; on one occasion, he rode seventy miles to a ranch in Wyoming, treated the rancher's gunshot wounds, and rode back to Billings within forty-eight hours. Many of the doctors who settled in Billings were well trained in eastern or midwestern cities; a few were Canadians.[17] Some Billings area doctors attended post-graduate medical schools in Chicago or New York to keep their medical knowledge current. Dr. Rosten Redd came to Miles City near Fort Keogh in 1881 after ten years experience as an army surgeon. It was said that he would ride a hundred miles to attend a patient, operating on the kitchen table under whiskey "anesthesia" with a butcher knife and common saw. Redd traveled to New York in 1885 for a year of advanced studies at Bellevue, St. Luke's, and Women's Hospitals. As county physician for the Yellowstone area, he performed, with the assistance of an army surgeon, a bilateral amputation for frozen

---

13 Ibid., 378-80.
14 Ibid., 52-53.
15 Sheila M. Rothman, *Living in the Shadow of Death: Tuberculosis and the Social Experience of Illness in American History* (Baltimore: Johns Hopkins University Press,1994), 161-75.
16 Robert F. Karolevitz, *Doctors of the Old West: A Pictorial History of Medicine on the Frontier* (New York: Bonanza Books: 1967), 47.
17 Phillips, *Medicine in the Making of Montana*, 389-92.

feet; the operation was reported in the *Yellowstone Journal* as "perfect in every respect."[18]

In 1879, a handful of physicians from various cities met in Helena, some two hundred miles from Billings, to organize a territorial medical association, later the Montana Medical Association. It was decided that the official organ of the society would be the *Medical Sentinel*, published from 1893 in Portland, Oregon.[19] The first hospital in Billings was not established until 1899, when the Sisters of Charity of Leavenworth, Kansas, supported by public subscription, opened St. Vincent's Hospital with space for fifty patients.[20]

In 1896, Montana, with a total population of some one hundred and thirty thousand (including less than one thousand Native-Americans), had close to two hundred and fifty physicians. This number included regular and sectarian practitioners. Six physicians including Townsend (all regulars) were listed for Billings in the 1896 *Medical and Surgical Register of the United States*. The population of the city at the time was a mere sixteen hundred, but the city's physicians probably covered sizeable outlying areas.[21]

Townsend established a medical practice in Billings, shortly after arriving.[22] In 1898, he was listed in the state gazetteer as "physician and coroner."[23] His reputation grew quickly. In his decade of practice in Montana, Townsend built statewide connections in the medical community and was lauded as "one of the oldest and most successful practitioners in Billings."[24] Despite his active

---

[18]   Ibid.,. 383-98. According to Phillips, the amputation by Redd was reported in the *Yellowstone Journal*, 24 December 1887; 383, 397.

[19]   Ibid., 405, 411.

[20]   St. Vincent's Hospital, Billings, MT website; http://www.svh-mt.org/body.cfm?id=55 (accessed July 2, 2010).

[21]   R.L. Polk, ed., *Medical and Surgical Register of the United States* (Detroit, Chicago: R.L. Polk & Co., 1896), 891-2.

[22]   Ibid., 892; Townsend is listed in the 1894-5 State Gazetteer; *Montana State Gazetteer and Business Directory*, 1681; photocopy courtesy Montana State Historical Society.

[23]   *Montana State Gazetteer and Business Directory* (1898), 1812; photocopy courtesy Montana State Historical Society.

[24]   "Obituary" (Ellis P. Townsend), *Medical Sentinel* 15 (1907): 454.

participation in the Medical Society of New Jersey, Townsend did not join the Montana Medical Association during his years of practice in that state.[25]

At some point in his first few years in Montana, he became surgeon of the Burlington Railway in Billings, a post that would have entailed the provision of medical services for train workers and building crews. This was almost certainly a part-time contract position.[26] Railway companies were among the first to set up hospitals and provide company-sponsored healthcare for their employees. The Northern Pacific, for example, opened a hospital in Missoula, Montana, in 1884 at a cost of $14,000.[27] Despite his editorial experience, Townsend did not become involved in an editorial capacity with the *Medical Sentinel*, which was published in Portland, Oregon, from 1893. (The *Medical Sentinel* listed contributing editors across several states.) His sole contribution to the journal was his article on "Back Alley Obstetrics," based on his past obstetrical experience in New Jersey.[28] Townsend also took on some military duties in 1898, perhaps examining local Montana recruits during the Spanish-American War or attending men on army posts.[29] The *Medical Sentinel* also took note of his amateur meteorological observations for the United States Weather Bureau in Billings.[30]

In 1901, Townsend was appointed government physician to the Crow Agency, a reservation about forty miles east of Billings.[31] His subsequent appointment to the Lame Deer Indian Reservation, an agency of the Northern Cheyenne administration located about one hundred miles east of Billings, was made in 1901, when he

---

[25]   Search of Montana Medical Association records from 1890 to 1910 courtesy Montana State Historical Society.

[26]   "Personals," *Medical Sentinel* 9 (1901): 398.

[27]   Karolevitz, *Doctors of the Old West*, 121.

[28]   EPT, "Back Alley Obstetrics," *Medical Sentinel* 2 (1894): 124-26. As noted previously, Townsend may have practiced in Philadelphia between 1884 and 1845; some of his obstetrical cases may have been in Philadelphia.

[29]   Camden County Medical Society, *History of the Camden County Medical Society, 1846-1956* (Camden: Camden County Medical Society, 1957), 143.

[30]   "Personals," *Medical* Sentinel 6 (1898): 118.

[31]   "Personals," *Medical Sentinel* 9 (1901): 398.

was sixty-six years old.[32] The *Billings' City Directory* for 1903-4 lists Townsend, with no local address and a note that he (and presumably his wife and children) had "moved to Lame Deer, Mont."[33] He was well regarded in Forsyth, a town thirty miles north of Lame Deer, where the weekly *Forsyth Times* later remembered him as a "Grand Old Man."[34] It is possible that Townsend resided in Forsyth or that he covered considerable distances responding to medical calls in the white as well as the Indian communities. His resignation in February, 1907, was listed in the *Indian School Journal* in April of that year. [35] His teenaged son, Edward Grubb Townsend, was listed as a clerk at the Tongue River Agency (which included the Lame Deer Reservation) and resigned in January, 1907, during his father's final illness.[36]

It is not difficult to imagine the hardships faced by a lone physician—an elderly man at that—in remote areas during the Montana winter. Townsend's death on July 30, 1907 at the age of

---

[32]   Townsend is listed among the white employees of the Indian Agency Service as a physician for the Tongue River Agency of Montana. His salary was $1000 in 1904 and $1200 in 1905. Tongue River is about one hundred and twenty miles northeast of Billings and may have been the original regional administrative center for the Lame Deer agency. Lame Deer is bounded on one side by the Tongue River. *Annual Reports of the Office of the Interior for the Fiscal Year Ending June 30th, 1905; Report of the Commissioner of Indian Affairs, Part 1* (Washington: Government Printing Office, 1906), 535; online at http://books.google.com/book s?id=49oRAAAAYAAJ&pg=PA535&dq=ellis+p+townsend+%22tongue+river%22&hl =en&ei=7FUyTPD2MYGClAf3nozACw&sa=X&oi=book_result&ct=result&resnum= 1&ved=0CCgQ6AEwAA#v=onepage&q=ellis%20p%20townsend%20%22tongue%20 river%22&f=false (accessed July 2, 2010). René Delaney drew my attention to these digitized agency reports.

[33]   *Billing's City Directory* (1903-4), 145; photocopy courtesy Montana State Historical Society.

[34]   *Forsyth Times*, August 1, 1907; photocopy courtesy Montana State Historical Society.

[35]   "Official Report of Indian Service Changes for February," *Indian School Journal* 7 (April 1907): 39, http://books.google.com/books?id=VGTXAAAAMAAJ&printsec=fro ntcover&dq=indian+school+journal&source=bl&ots=o30x_q3UpS&sig=fnJX_sus-5-O ysLpL5s9NbAevwM&hl=en&ei=h01rTPnmKoXGlQen0LiSAQ&sa=X&oi=book_result &ct=result&resnum=1&ved=0CBoQ6AEwAA#v=onepage&q&f=false (accessed July 2, 2010).

[36]   "Official Report of Indian Service Changes for January," *Indian School Journal* 7 (March 1907): 71.

seventy-two was indeed tragic.[37] Amputations for frostbite were a familiar theme in Montana's medical history. For example, in 1862, Dr. George Hamilton, surgeon to a railroad scouting expedition and later attached to Fort Owen, successfully amputated the legs of a man suffering from frostbite. But this time the victim was the physician himself. The headline in the *Billings Daily Gazette* for July 31, 1907, told the story: "Dr. Townsend Answers Call: Death Summons Well Known Billings Physician—Exposure Was To [sic] Much—Had Both Feet Frozen Last Winter While Making a Call to Lame Deer Agency and Shock Following Caused Gradual Decline:"

> Last winter the doctor was unusually exposed to the elements, while answering a call near Lame Deer, where he was employed as government physician, and his last illness was the result of that exposure. At the time he froze both of his feet and it was found necessary to amputate several of his toes. When first taken sick he was taken to the hospital [probably St. Vincent Hospital in Billings], but later removed to his home. Being of an advanced age, he was unable to withstand the long sickness and gradually grew worse until the end.[38]

The exact nature of Townsend's decline was unclear, but it is probable that he died of the debilitating effects of gangrene and chronic infection in his feet and legs—a painful and difficult death in those pre-antibiotic days. The *Journal of the American Medical Association* published a brief obituary for Townsend, probably reported to the *Journal* by a Montana colleague and drawing on Townsend's registration information in Association files. It was remarked in that obituary that Townsend had suffered amputation of his feet, suggesting more extensive gangrene than involvement of the toes alone.[39] While not placing too much reliance on these press reports as medical documents, the

37   Confirmed by Montana Office of Vital Statistics, *Montana Death Index, 1907-2002*; index number 01-0350. Photocopy, courtesy Montana State Historical Society.
38   "Dr. Townsend Answers Call," *Billings Daily Gazette*, July 31, 1907, p. 3.
39   "Ellis P. Townsend," Obituary, *Journal of the American Medical Association* 49 (1907): 710.

discrepancies might reflect a two-stage amputation as infection or gangrene progressed.

In the local newspaper, Townsend was hailed as a "pioneer resident" and "one of the ablest physicians and surgeons in the state."[40] The press in Forsyth, a town relatively close to the Lame Deer agency, remembered him as "well-known in this country." He was eulogized as a doctor who had "sacrificed his life in allaying the sufferings of others."[41] He is buried in the Mountainview Cemetery in Billings.[42] The old New Jersey doctors would have called Townsend a "martyr to his profession," a term often applied in nineteenth-century medical society obituaries to brother physicians who died of tuberculosis or other afflictions acquired in the course of attending a patient.

---

[40] "Dr. Townsend Answers Call," *Billings Daily Gazette,* July 31, 1907.

[41] *Forsyth Times*, August 8, 1907, n.p. Photocopy, courtesy Montana State Historical Society.

[42] Corky Knebel, "T Index for Mountainview Cemetery, Billings, MT.," United States GenWeb Archives, *http://files.usgwarchives.org/mt/yellowstone/cemeteries/mtview/t. txt* (accessed July 2, 2010).

AFTERWORD

In the two years of its existence, the *Country Practitioner*, Ellis P. Townsend's brave little journal, addressed many of the themes of nineteenth-century American medicine and medical practice. From the Civil War until his death in 1907, Townsend lived a quintessentially American medical life—perhaps a bit longer on adventure that many of his colleagues. Though long forgotten and difficult to find in libraries and archives, the *Country Practitioner* has earned a place in the history of medicine in late-nineteenth-century New Jersey and in the broader spectrum of American medical journalism. In a state with few medical publications, the *Country Practitioner; Or New Jersey Journal of Medical & Surgical Practice*, shone brightly, if briefly. And none can deny that it was, as historian David Cowen wrote, a "lively" little journal.

BIBLIOGRAPHY

Multiple publications by a single author are listed chronologically. Membership rosters of county medical societies were published in the *TMSNJ*; there are referenced in the footnotes and are not included in the bibliography. All references from the *Country Practitioner* are listed in a separate section following the general bibliography.

Abbreviation: *Transactions of the Medical Society of New Jersey*: *TMSNJ*

GENERAL BIBLIOGRAPHY

"Addison W. Taylor" (obituary). *Journal of the Medical Society of New Jersey* 1 (1904-1905): 161.

American Medical Association. *Code of Medical Ethics of the American Medical Association.* Chicago: American Medical Association Press, 1847. http://www.ama-assn.org/ama1/pub/upload/mm/369/1847code.pdf (accessed 2 July 2010).

American Medical Association. *Directory of Deceased American Physicians.* Chicago: American Medical Association, 1993.

Annual Reports of the Office of the Interior for the Fiscal Year Ending June 30th, 1905; Report of the Commissioner of Indian Affairs, Part 1. Washington: Government Printing Office, 1906. http://books.google.com/books?id=49o RAAAAYAAJ&pg=PA535&dq=ellis+p+townsend+%22tongue+river%22&hl= en&ei=7FUyTPD2MYGClAf3nozACw&sa=X&oi=book_result&ct=result&re snum=1&ved=0CCgQ6AEwAA#v=onepage&q=ellis%20p%20townsend%20 %22tongue%20river%22&f=false (accessed July 2, 2010).

Bateman, R.M. "Mental Pathology and Criminal Law." *TMSNJ* (1876): 76-95.

Beasley, Henry. *The Book of Prescriptions*. Philadelphia: Lindsay & Blakiston, 1857.

Beverly Weekly Visitor. Beverly, NJ: 1877-9 with gaps. Microfilm, Rutgers University Libraries, New Brunswick, NJ.

Billing's City Directory (1903-4), 14.

Billings, John Shaw. "Literature and Institutions." In Edward H. Clarke, Henry J. Bigelow, Samuel D. Gross, T. Gaillard Thomas, J.S. Billings. *A Century of American Medicine 1776-1876*, 291-366. Philadelphia: Henry C. Lea, 1876. Reprint, New York: Burt Franklin, 1971.

_____. "The Medical Journals of the United States." *Boston Medical and Surgical Journal* 100 (1879): 1-14.

Biographical Review, Volume XIX, Containing Life Sketches of Leading Citizens of Burlington and Camden Counties, New Jersey. Boston: Biographical Review Publishing Company, 1897.

W.M. Brown. "Reports of District Societies: Essex County." *TMSNJ* (1863): 53-56.

"Buchanan Gives Up the Fight: Charters of Two of the Bogus Medical Colleges Annulled." *New York Times*, October 1, 1880.

Burlington County Hospital Board of Managers. *Sixth Annual Report of the Board of Managers of Burlington County Hospital, Mt. Holly*, 1866. Special Collections and University Archives, Rutgers University, New Brunswick, NJ.

Burlington County Medical Society Minute Book: 1869-1893. Burlington County Medical Society Records, University of Medicine and Dentistry of New Jersey Special Collections, Newark, NJ.

Butler, Samuel W., ed. *The Medical Register and Directory of the United States*. Philadelphia: Office of the Medical and Surgical Reporter, 1878.

Camden County Medical Society. *History of the Camden County Medical Society, 1846-1956*. Camden: Camden County Medical Society, 1957.

Chapman, Carleton B. *Order Out of Chaos: John Shaw Billings and America's Coming of Age*. Boston: Boston Medical Library, 1994.

Clark, J. Henry. "The First Fifty Years of the District Medical Society of Essex County." *TMSNJ* (1867): 77-185.

[Coleman, J.P.?]. "Reports of District Societies, Burlington County." *TMSNJ* (1866): 150.

Coleman, J.P. "Reports of District Societies: Burlington County." *TMSNJ* (1869): 115-16.

Cowen, David L. *Medicine and Health in New Jersey: A History*. Princeton: D. Van Nostrand, 1964.

Craig, Neville B. *Recollections of an Ill-Fated Expedition to the Headwaters of the Madeira River in Brazil*. Philadelphia: J.B. Lippincott, 1907. http://books.google.com/books, enter "Recollections of an Ill-Fated Voyage" (accessed July 2, 2010).

Cramer, Richard. "Ellis P. Townsend: 1835-1907." Genealogy.com website. http://genforum.genealogy.com/townsend/messages/481.html (accessed 2 July 2010).

Delaney, René. "Genealogy: Ellis P. Townsend + Almira Jennie Johnston." PhpGedView website. http://renesfamily.com/family/family.php?famid=F00439&ged=Renes.GED and http://renesfamily.com/family/individual.php?pid=I01010&ged=Renes.GED (accessed July 2, 2010).

DePalma, Ralph G., Virginia W. Hayes, and Leo R. Zacharski. "Bloodletting: Past and Present." *Journal of the American College of Surgeons* 205 (2007): 132-44.

"Dr. Townsend Answers Call," *Billings Daily Gazette*, July 31, 1907.

"Ellis P. Townsend" (obituary). *Journal of the American Medical Association* 49 (1907): 710.

"Expedition to Brazil." *New York Times*, January 3, 1878.

Forsyth Times, Forsyth, MT, August 1, 1907; August 8, 1907 (untitled obituary and funeral notice for Ellis P. Townsend).

"Funeral Rites Held for Power Official" (Edward Grubb Townsend). *Billings Gazette*, March 26, 1947.

Fye, W. Bruce. "The Literature of American Internal Medicine: A Historical View." *Annals of Internal Medicine* 196 (1987): 451-60.

_____. "Medical Authorship: Traditions, Trends, and Tribulations." *Annals of Internal Medicine* 113 (1990): 317-325.

Gardner, Joel R. *Neighbor Caring for Neighbor: The History of the Medical Staff, Memorial Hospital of Burlington County, 1880-1995*. Burlington, NJ: Memorial Health Alliance, ca.1996.

"General E. Burd Grubb Dies in 72d Year," *New York Times*, July 8, 1913, p. 7.

Godfrey, E.L.B. *History of the Medical Profession of Camden County, New Jersey*. Camden: F.A. Davis, 1896.

Goodman, Louis S. and Alfred Gilman. *The Pharmacological Basis of Therapeutics*. 2nd ed. New York: Macmillan, 1955.

Gross, Samuel D. "Surgery" In Edward H. Clarke, Henry J. Bigelow, Samuel D. Gross, T. Gaillard Thomas, J.S. Billings. *A Century of American Medicine 1776-1876*, 115-215. Philadelphia: Henry C. Lea, 1876. Reprint, New York: Burt Franklin, 1971.

Holmes, Oliver Wendell. "On the Contagiousness of Puerperal Fever." Paper read at the Boston Society for Medical Improvement in 1843 and published in the *New England Quarterly Journal for Medicine and Surgery 1 (1843)*. http://www.bartleby.com/38/5/1.html; accessed July 2, 2010.

_____. "On the Contagiousness of Puerperal Fever" (selected passages). In *Source Book of Medical History*, edited by Logan Clendening, 603-6. New York: Henry Schuman, 1942. Reprint New York: Dover, 1960.

Howard-Jones, Norman. "A Critical Study of the Origins and Early Development of Hypodermic Medication." *Journal of the History of Medicine and the Allied Sciences* 2 (1947): 201-48.

Howell, Joel D. *Technology in the Hospital: Transforming Patient Care in the Early Twentieth Century.* Baltimore: Johns Hopkins University Press, 1995.

Hunt, Ezra Mundy. "Origin of Disease and Micro-Organisms as Related Thereto," *TMSNJ* (1888): 95-111.

Karolevitz, Robert F. *Doctors of the Old West: A Pictorial History of Medicine on the Frontier.* New York: Bonanza Books, 1967.

Keating, John M. *How to Examine for Life Insurance.* Philadelphia: W.B. Saunders, 1891.

Knebel, Corky. "T index for Mountainview Cemetery, Billings, MT." United States GenWeb Archives. *http://files.usgwarchives.org/mt/yellowstone/ cemeteries/mtview/t.txt* (accessed July 2, 2010).

Library of the Surgeon-General's Office. *Index-Catalogue of the Library of the Surgeon-General's Office Library*, Series 1. Washington: Government Printing Office, 1880. http://indexcat.nlm.nih.gov/ (accessed July 2, 2010).

Marks, Harry H. *The Progress of Experiment: Science and Therapeutic Reform in the United States: 1900-1990.* Cambridge: Cambridge University Press, 1997.

Medical Directory of Philadelphia, Pennsylvania, and Delaware and the Southern Half of New Jersey. Philadelphia: P. Blakiston, 1885.

Montana Office of Vital Statistics. *Montana Death Index, 1907-2002*; index number 01-0350.

Montana State Gazetteer and Business Directory (1894-5), 1681; (1898): 1812.

Moss, Sandra W. "The Most Dreaded Complication of Labor: The Early Treatment of Eclampsia in New Jersey." *New Jersey Medicine* 98 (April 2001): 43-48.

_____. "James Still and the Regulars: The Struggle for Legitimacy." *New Jersey Medicine* 98 (October 2001): 39-44.

_____. "The Power to Terrify: Eclampsia in Nineteenth-Century American Practice." *Journal of Obstetrical, and Gynecologic, and Neonatal Nursing* 31 (2002): 514-20.

_____. "The Doctor as Weatherman: Medical Topography in Nineteenth-Century New Jersey." *Journal of the Rutgers University Libraries* 62 (2006): 59-74. http://jrul.libraries.rutgers.edu (accessed July 2, 2010).

_____. "This Destroying Scourge: Yellow Fever Epidemics of the 1790s in New Jersey." *New Jersey Heritage* 5 (2006): 10-23.

_____. "Fountains of Youth: New Jersey Water-Cures," *Garden State Legacy* 1(2) (2008), online at GardenStateLegacy.com (access limited to subscribers).

National Park Service. "Camp Letterman General Hospital." http://www.nps. gov/archive/gett/getttour/sidebar/letterman.htm (accessed July 2, 2010)

New Jersey State Data Center. "New Jersey Resident Population by County: 1880-1920." In *New Jersey Population Trends: 1790-2000* (Trenton: New Jersey Department of Labor, 2001), 23, http://lwd.dol.state.nj.us/labor/lpa/ census/2kpub/njsdcp3.pdf (accessed August 26, 2010).

"Obituary" (Ellis P. Townsend). *Medical Sentinel* 15(1907): 454.

Office of the Surgeon General. *Medical and Surgical History of the War of the Rebellion*. Washington: Government Printing Office, 1870-1888. Reprinted with editorial additions, Wilmington NC: Broadfoot Publishing Co., 1990.

"Official Report of Indian Service Changes for February." *Indian School Journal* 7 (March 1907): 71 (April 1907): 39. http://books.google.com/books?id=V GTXAAAAMAAJ&printsec=frontcover&dq=indian+school+journal&source =bl&ots=o30x_q3UpS&sig=fnJX_sus-5-OysLpL5s9NbAevwM&hl=en&ei=h0 1rTPnmKoXGlQen0LiSAQ&sa=X&oi=book_result&ct=result&resnum=1&v ed=0CBoQ6AEwAA#v=onepage&q&f=false (accessed July 2, 2010).

Osler, William. *Principles and Practice of Medicine*. 3rd ed. New York: D. Appleton, 1898.

Paragraph Club. *Beverly: A Local History*. Beverly, NJ: Paragraph Club and Beverly Bicentennial Committee, 1977.

Parrish, Joseph. "Historical Address." In Burlington County Medical Society. *Semi-Centennial Anniversary of the District Medical Society for the County of Burlington, June 17*, 5-30. Beverly, NJ: Banner Steam-Power Print: 1879.

Peitzman, Steven J. "'Thoroughly Practical': America's Polyclinic Medical Schools," *Bulletin of the History of Medicine* 54 (1980): 166-87.

"Personals." *Medical Sentinel* 6 (1898): 118.

"Personals." *Medical Sentinel* 9 (1901): 398.

Phillips, Paul C. *Medicine in the Making of Montana*. Missoula: Montana State University Press, 1962.

Pierson, William. "Minutes: One Hundred and Tenth Annual Meeting, Medical Society of New Jersey." *TMSNJ* (1876): 15-29.

Pierson, William. "Transactions of the Medical Society of New Jersey: The One Hundred and Twenty-Third Annual Meeting." *TMSNJ* (1889), 23-43.

_____. "Transactions of the Medical Society of New Jersey: The One Hundred and Twenty-Fourth Annual Meeting." *TMSNJ* (1890): 23-75.

_____. "Transactions of the Medical Society of New Jersey: The One Hundred and Twenty-Fifth Annual Meeting." *TMSNJ* (1891): 23-51.

Polk, R.L., ed. *Medical and Surgical Register of the United States*. 4th rev. ed. Detroit: R.L. Polk & Co., 1896.

Purdy, Alfred E.M. succeeded by Wm. H. White, eds. *The Medical Registry of New York, New Jersey, and Connecticut*. New York: G.P. Putnam's Sons, issued annually during the 1870 and 1880s.

"Regular Physicians in New Jersey: 1866." *TMSNJ* (1866): 313.

"Repeal of Charter of the Medical and Surgical College of New Jersey—New Jersey State Board of Medical Examiners." *Boston Medical and Surgical Journal* 124 (1891): 299.

Rogers, Fred B. and A. Reasoner Sayre. *The Healing Art: A History of the Medical Society of New Jersey, 1766-1966*. Trenton, NJ: Medical Society of New Jersey, 1966.

Rosenberg, Charles E. "Making It in Urban Medicine: A Career in the Age of Scientific Medicine." In *Explaining Epidemics and Other Studies in the History of Medicine*, 215-42. Cambridge: Cambridge University Press, 1992.

Rothman, Sheila M. *Living in the Shadow of Death: Tuberculosis and the Social Experience of Illness in American History*. Baltimore: Johns Hopkins University Press, 1994.

Rothstein, William G. *American Physicians in the Nineteenth Century: From Sects to Science*. Baltimore: Johns Hopkins University Press, 1985.

Rutkow, Ira. *American Surgery: An Illustrated History*. Philadelphia: Lippincott-Raven, 1998.

Sabin, Florence Rena. *Franklin Paine Mall—The Story of a Mind*. Baltimore: Johns Hopkins University Press, 1934.

Saint Vincent Hospital, Billings, MT. http://www.svh-mt.org/body.cfm?id=55 (accessed July 2, 2010).

Secretary's Book: Burlington County Medical Society, 1829-1866, Burlington Country Medical Society Records. University Libraries Special Collections, University of Medicine and Dentistry of New Jersey, Newark, NJ.

Shaw, W.H. "Beverly Township and City." In *History of Burlington and Mercer Counties*, edited by E.M. Woodward and John F. Hageman, 231-47. Philadelphia: Everts and Peck, 1883.

Sherk, Henry H. *Colleagues and Competitors: A Sesquicentennial History of the Camden County Medical Society: 1846-1996*. Voorhees, NJ: Camden Country Medical Society, 1996.

Shorter, Edward. *From Paralysis to Fatigue*. New York: Free Press, 1992.

[Shrady, George]. "The Country Practitioner." *Medical Record New York* 3 (1868): 229-30.

Snape, William J. "The Rise and Fall of John Buchanan 'M.D.': Founder of Livingstone University, Haddonfield, N.J." *Bulletin of the Camden County Historical Society* 24 (1970): 17-9.

Snowden, John W. [as Jno. W.]. "Reports of District Societies: Camden County." *TMSNJ* (1884): 192-97.

————. "Reports of District Societies: Camden County." TMSNJ (1887): 310-18.

Stevenson, John R. "A History of Medicine and Medical Men." In *A History of the Camden County Medical and Surgical Society*, edited by George R. Prowell, 237-308. Philadelphia: L.J. Richards, 1886.

Still, James. *Early Recollections and Life of James Still*. Philadelphia: J.B. Lippincott, 1877.

Strock, Daniel. "Reports of District Societies: Camden County." *TMSNJ* (1893): 209.

Taylor, H. Genet. "Report of the Delegate to the Pennsylvania State Medical Society." *TMSNJ* (1879): 34.

Thornton, S.C. "Reports of District Societies: Burlington County." *TMSNJ* (1871): 253-57.

Thornton, S.C. "Reports of District Societies: Burlington County," *TMSNJ* (1873): 129-35.

Thornton, S.C. "Reports of District Societies: Burlington Country." *TMSNJ* (1875): 113-16.

Townsend, Ellis P. "Special Cases by Dr. E.P. Townsend." *TMSNJ* (1866): 158-61.

_____. "Tabular Statement of Diseases Occurring in the Practice of Dr. E.P. Townsend, Beverly, NJ. January, 1868 to January, 1869." *TMSNJ* (1869): 126.

_____. "Cases by Dr. Townsend:Obstetrics," *TMSNJ* (1873): 135-37.

_____. *Suburban Homes.* (ca. 1874). Burlington County Historical Society, Burlington, NJ.

_____. "Case of Chronic Splenitis." *TMSNJ* (1876): 116-19.

_____. "Communication by Dr. Townsend." *TMSNJ* (1876): 181-83.

_____. "Medical Heroism." *TMSNJ* (1876): 96-101.

_____. "Report of Delegate to State Medical Society of Pennsylvania." *TMSNJ* (1880): 32-3.

_____. "Reports of District Societies: Camden County." *TMSNJ* (1888), 181-88.

_____. "Reports of District Societies: Camden County." *TMSNJ* (1889): 183-89.

_____. "Reports of District Societies: Camden County." *TMSNJ* (1891), 268-74.

_____. "Reports of District Societies: Camden County." *TMSNJ* (1892), 236-38.

_____. "Back Alley Obstetrics." *Medical Sentinel* 2 (1894): 124-6.

United States Bureau of the Census (1880). Population of the 100 Largest Urban Places." *http://www.census.gov/population/www/documentation/twps0027/tab11.txt* (accessed July 2, 2010).

Wade, Nancy M. "Historic Homes and Genealogy." in *Beverly: A Local History*, edited by Paragraph Club, 112-50. Beverly NJ: Paragraph Club and Bicentennial Committee, 1977.

Wagner, C[linton]. *Report of Interesting Surgical Operations Performed at the U.S.A. General Hospital, Beverly, New Jersey.* 1865. Photocopy courtesy American Philosophical Society, Philadelphia.

Wagner, Frederick B., Jr. and J. Woodrow Savacool, eds. *Jefferson History: Thomas Jefferson University: A Chronological History and Alumni Directory, 1824-1990.* Philadelphia: Thomas Jefferson University, 1992. *http://jdc.jefferson.edu/cgi/viewcontent.cgi?article=1032&context=wagner1* (accessed 2 July 2010).

Warner, John Harley. "From Specificity to Universalism in Medical Therapeutics: Transformation in 19th-Century United States." In *Sickness and Health in America: Readings in the History of Medicine and Public Health.* 3rd ed. Edited by Judith Walzer Leavitt and Ronald L. Numbers, 87-101. Madison, WI: University of Wisconsin Press, 1997.

_____. *The Therapeutic Perspective: Medical Practice, Knowledge, and Identity in America, 1820-1885.* Princeton: Princeton University Press: 1997.

Wickes, Stephen, ed. *The Rise, Minutes, and Proceedings of the New Jersey Medical Society, Established July 23rd, 1766.* Newark: Jennings and Hardham, 1875.

Williams, John Whitridge. "Medical Education and the Midwife Problem." *Journal of the American Medical Association* 58 (1912): 1-7.

Wilmarth, Frank. "Reports of District Societies: Essex County." *TMSNJ* (1874): 131-38.

Wood, George B. and Franklin Bache. *Dispensatory of the United States of America*. Philadelphia: Lippincott, 1883.

Yoka, Stanley and Ethel Salamone. "Bits of the Past," In *Beverly: A Local History*, edited by Paragraph Club, 237-88. Beverly NJ: Paragraph Club and Bicentennial Committee, 1977.

Young, Irene Dupont. *Obstetric Register* (1849-1880). University of Medicine and Dentistry of New Jersey Special Collections, Newark, NJ.

COUNTRY PRACTITIONER BIBLIOGRAPHY

Titled and untitled editorials written but unsigned by Townsend are indicated as [Townsend, Ellis P.]. Issue numbers and month of publication are indicated for all *Country Practitioner* entries in the bibliography.

Abbreviation: *Country Practitioner*: *CP*

Barnes. "General Conclusions in Regard to the Use of Forceps." *CP* 1, no. 6 (November 1879): 248. Reprinted from *Obstetrical Journal*, no further citation.

Bartholow, Roberts. "On the Therapeutics of Acute Rheumatism." *CP* 1, no. 10 (March 1880): 325-31. Reprinted from *Medical News and Abstract*, no further citation.

"Clergymen in the Sick Room." *CP* 2, no. 1 (June 1880): 29-30. Reprinted from the *Chicago Medical Gazette*, no further citation.

"The Clergy Must Pay." *CP* 1, no. 12 (May 1880): 433-34. Reprinted from *Chicago Medical Gazette*, no further citation.

Corson, Hiram. "Post-partum Binders." *CP* 2, no. 5 (October 1880): 149-52.

_____. "On Small-Pox." *CP* 3, no. 3 (September 1881): 81-86.

"Country versus City Practice." *CP* 1, no. 3 (August 1879): 134-35. Reprinted from *Medical and Surgical Reporter*, no further citation.

"Domestic Department: Why Women Fade." *CP* 3, no. 1 (July 1881): 14-16. Reprinted from *Good Health*, no further citation.

"Domestic Department: Sleeplessness from Thought." *CP* 2, no. 12 (May, 1881): 402-4. Reprinted from Grandville, "Common Mind Troubles," no further citation.

"Domestic Department: Weary Women." *CP* 2, no. 12 (May, 1881): 404-5. Reprinted from *Sanitary Magazine*, no further citation.

Elwell, Alexander. "Should We Bandage after Labor and Why?" *CP* 1, no. 12 (May 1880): 417-19.

Gross, Samuel D. "A Discourse on Bloodletting Considered as a Therapeutic Agent." *CP* 2, nos. 10, 11 (March, April 1881): 337-45, 371-78.

Gross, Samuel D. "Correspondence." *CP* 2, no. 10 (March 1881): 330-31.

Heritage, J. Down. "Clinical Reports in Private Practice." *CP* 1, no. 11 (April 1880): 361-70.

Heritage, J. Down. "The Medical Profession." *CP* 2, no. 2 (July 1880): 40-42.

Hickman, J.W. "The Value of Experience in the Practice of Medicine." *CP*, 1, no. 8 (January 1880): 253-55.

Howe, A.J. "When Obstetrical Forceps Are to Be Used." *CP* 2, no. 12 (May 1881): 416-17. Reprinted from the *American Medical Journal*, St. Louis, no further citation.

Jones, H. Webster. "Obstetric Aphorisms." *CP* 3, no. 3 (September 1881): 115-16.

Jacobi, Abraham. "Dr. A. Jacobi Says," *CP* 2, no. 9 (February 1881): 318. Reprinted from *New York Medical Record*, no further citation.

Lapian, S.Q. "Letter to the Editor." *CP* 1, no. 3 (August, 1879): 87-90.

"List of Physicians." *CP* 2, no. 3 (August 1881): 79-80.

Mann, Edward C. "Mental Responsibility and the Diagnosis of Insanity in Criminal Cases." *CP* 1, no. 2 (July, 1879): 10-20.

Michener, E. "Notes on Bloodletting as a Remedy." *CP*, 2, no. 9 (February1881): 289-92.

Mitchell, S. Weir. "Neurasthenia, Hysteria, and Their Treatment." *CP* 2, no. 1 (July 1879): 19-22. Reprinted from the *Chicago Medical Gazette*, no further citation.

"On Veratrum Viride." *CP* 1, no. 1 (June 1879): 22-23.

Page, R.H. "Report of Case from *Transactions of the Burlington County Medical Society*." *CP* 2, no. 1 (June 1880): 1-6.

Parrish, Joseph. "Historical Address: Semi-Centennial Meeting of the Burlington County Medical Society." *CP* 1, no. 2 (July 1879: Supplement): 4-20, with introductory remarks 1-3.

Sigsbee, W. "On Veratrum Viride." *CP* 1, no. 1 (June 1879): 22. Reprinted from the *Medical and Surgical Reporter*, no further citation.

Stauffer, S.S, "The Country Medical Practitioner in Contrast with the City Practitioner." *CP* 1, no. 10 (March 1880): 333-35.

T. [Townsend, Ellis P.?] "Leaves from the Diary of a Country Doctor." *CP* 2, no. 12 (May 1881): 395-97.

Townsend, Ellis P. "Puerperal Eclampsia." *CP* 1, no. 2 (July 1879): 26-28.

_____. "New Jersey State Medical Society." *CP* 2, no. 1 (June 1880): 11-12.

_____. "Medical Practice in Brazil." *CP* 2, no. 3 (August 1880): 75-77.

_____. "Our Subscribers." *CP* 2, no. 3 (August 1880): 105.

_____. "Sick Room Visitations." *CP* 2, no. 6 (November 1880): 191-92.

_____. "An Artful Dodger." *CP* 2, no. 9 (February 1881): 294-95.

_____. "Double Pneumonia: Clinical Report of a Typical Case of Pneumonia." *CP* 2, no. 10 (March 1881): 323-26.

[Townsend, Ellis P.]. "To Medical Practitioners." *CP* 1, no. 1 (June 1879): 1-3.

_____. "New Remedies" *CP* 1, no 1 (June 1879): 33. ??SIGNED

_____. "Editorial," *CP* 1, no. 3 (August 1879): 106.

_____. "Editorial," *CP* 1, no. 3 (August 1879): 107.

_____. "Editorial," *CP* 1, no. 4 (September 1879): 141.

_____. "Editorial," *CP* 1, no. 4 (September 1879): 143.

_____. "Advertising Rates," *CP* 1, no. 6 (November 1879): 213.

_____. "Editorial," *CP* 1, no. 6 (November 1879): 213-15.

_____. "Editorial," *CP* 1, no. 7 (December 1879): 251.

_____. "City and Country Doctors." *CP* 1, no. 8 (January 1880): 258-61.

_____. "Gratuitous Services to Clergymen." *CP* 1, no 8 (January 1880): 264-65.

_____. "Please Answer the Following Questionnaire," *CP* 1, nos. 8,9 (January, February 1880): back covers.

_____. "Public Accommodations." *CP* 1, no. 11 (April 1880): 398.

_____. "Editorial," *CP* 1, no. 11 (April 1880): 399.

_____. "Editorial", *CP* 1, no. 12 (May 1880): 435-36.

_____. "Notes and Comments: Anaesthetics." *CP* 1, no. 12 (May 1880): 425-26.

_____. "Bogus Diplomas." *CP* 2, no. 1 (June 1880): 32-33.

_____. "Wanted—Backbone." *CP* 2, no. 5 (October 1880): 158.

_____. "Diet for the Sick." *CP* 2, no. 6 (November 1880), 192-93.

_____. "Personal," *CP* 2, no. 6), (November 1880): 211.

_____. "Editorial," *CP* 2 no. 7 (December 1880): 248.

_____. "Domestic Department: Popular Fallacies." *CP* 2, no. 8 (January 1881): 262-5. Sections reprinted from *Good Health*, no further citation.

_____. "Editorial," *CP* 2, no. 8 (January 1881): 285.

_____. "Editorial," *CP* 2, no. 10 (March 1881): 354.

_____. "Editorial," *CP* 2, no. 10 (March 1881): 353.

_____. "Leaves from the Diary of a Country Doctor," *CP* 2, no. 10 (March 1881): 326-30.

_____. "Practice Hunters." *CP* 2, no. 11 (April 1881): 366-67.

_____. "Editorial," *CP* 2, no. 11 (April 1881): 387-88.

_____. "Editorial," *CP* 2, no. 11 (April 1881): 388-89.

_____. "Editorial." *CP* 2, no. 12 (May 1881): 423.

_____. "Editorial,", *CP* 3, no. 1 (July 1881): 39.

_____. "Society Transactions: State Medical Society of New Jersey." *CP* 3, no. 1 (July 1881): 5-8.

_____. "Society Transactions: American Medical Association." *CP* 3, no. 1 (July 1881): 2-3.

_____. "Notes and Comments: Vaccination." *CP* 3, no. 3 (September 1881): 86-87.

_____. "Editorial" (Smallpox, followed by questionnaire). *CP* 3, no. 3 (September 1881): 116-18.

Townsend, W.W. "Propylamine Chloride in Acute Inflammatory Rheumatism." *CP* 1, no. 5 (October 1879):147-49.

"Treatment of the Drowned," *CP* 1, no. 6 (November 1879): 192-5. Reprinted from *Proceedings of the Medical Society, County of Kings*, which reprinted the article from the State Board of Health of Michigan, no further citations.

Watson. "Leaves from the Diary of a Country Doctor." *CP* 2, no. 11 (April 1881): 363-5.

Wilkerson, T.S. "Removal of Both Ovaria, or 'Battey's Operation' for the Cure of Insanity." *CP* 3, no. 2 (August 1881): 56-61.

INDEX